CONTEMPORARY CHALLENGES IN ENDOCARDITIS

Edited by **Michael S. Firstenberg**

Contemporary Challenges in Endocarditis
http://dx.doi.org/10.5772/62550
Edited by Michael S. Firstenberg

Contributors

Gregory Scalia, Cheima Wathek, Pedro Diz-Dios, Miguel Castro, Francisco-Javier Alvarez, Javier Fernandez-Feijoo, Marcio Diniz-Freitas, Lucia Garcia-Caballero, Jacobo Limeres, Marion Skalweit, Michael S Firstenberg, Fabian Giraldo, Héctor Rafael Díaz García, Nancy Anabel Contreras-De La Torre, Alfonso Alemán-Villalobos, María De Jesús Carrillo-Galindo, Olivia Berenice Gómez-Jiménez, Edgar Esparza-Beléndez, Gladys Eloísa Ramírez-Rosales, Eliseo Portilla- De Buen, Ramón Arreola-Torres, Stanislaw Stawicki

Published by InTech

Janeza Trdine 9, 51000 Rijeka, Croatia

Publishing Process Manager Iva Simcic

Technical Editor SPi Global

Cover InTech Design team

First published November, 2016

Printed in Croatia

Additional hard copies can be obtained from orders@intechopen.com

Contemporary Challenges in Endocarditis, Edited by Michael S. Firstenberg

p. cm.

Print ISBN 978-953-51-2769-7
Online ISBN 978-953-51-2770-3

Meet the editor

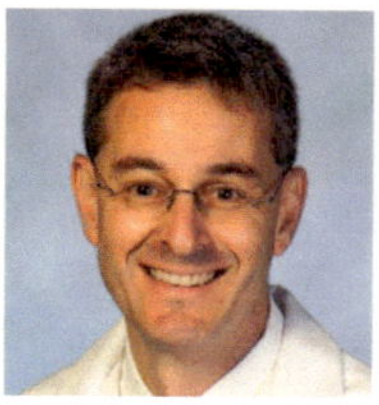

Dr. Michael S. Firstenberg is a board-certified thoracic surgeon actively practicing adult cardiac surgery at Summa Akron City Hospital in Akron, Ohio. He serves as an associate professor at Northeast Ohio Medical University. He attended Case Western Reserve University for Medical School, received his General Surgery training at the University Hospitals of Cleveland, and completed a Fellowship in Thoracic Surgery at the Ohio State University. He also obtained advanced training in heart failure surgical therapies at the Cleveland Clinic. He has lectured worldwide and written more than 100 peer-reviewed articles, several textbook chapters, and edited 3 books—including this update on endocarditis. In addition, he is active in numerous professional societies, clinical research projects, and various quality, process improvement, and multidisciplinary committees.

Contents

Preface

Endocarditis, by definition, represents an infection of the heart or, more specifically, the valves or intracardiac structures. The diagnosis and management of these complex infections have challenged clinicians for years—and despite significant advances, they continue to do so. The physiologic consequences of not only systemic sepsis from the bacteremia but sometimes, more importantly, also the associated acute congestive heart failure from involvement of the cardiac valves can be difficult to manage and potentially catastrophic in presentation. Overwhelming infections can also result in intracardiac fistulae with shunting and arrhythmias that can be difficult to manage and often are indications for emergent intervention. Coronary embolisms of infected material can further cloud the clinical picture as patients may present with signs and symptoms of an acute myocardial infarction. Nevertheless, there have been significant improvements in the initial diagnosis and management of these problems. A greater awareness of the presentations of sepsis and the recognition that a substantial subset of patients with complex comorbidities may have associated endocarditis have contributed to the greater recognition and incidence of this diagnosis. Furthermore, advances in diagnostic testing have allowed for more specific identification of causative agents as more and more patients present with polymicrobial infections, fungal infections, drug-resistant organisms, and even atypical or culture-negative endocarditis from noninfectious sources.

Without a doubt, the growing spectrum of comorbidities that patients present with places them at increased risk for developing these catastrophic infections. The dramatic increase in substance abuse, especially heroin and synthetic drugs, has also resulted in a significant increase in younger patients presenting with complex cardiac infections. Often, patients because of their physiologic reserve may not present until late in their clinical course with extremely challenging cardiopulmonary problems with potentially devastating septic emboli. Their socioeconomic and compliance problems combined with the mental health issues that are associated with drug abuse make this population extremely difficult to manage successfully both short term and long term. In addition, the growing use of intravascular and cardiac support devices such as pacemakers, defibrillators, left ventricular assist devices, intravascular ports, and long-term monitoring devices places patients at increased risk for infections that can be difficult to manage. Greater access to cardiac surgery with more patients getting either surgical or percutaneous valve procedures has also resulted in an increased incidence of infections. Furthermore, as patients develop more problems that historically might have limited their life span, combined with the growing use of immunomodulating medications for a variety of disorders, there is also an inherent increase of the risk for all types of infections—including endocarditis. It is becoming better understood that these populations, such as those with end-stage renal disease, require a greater index of suspicion with aggressive and timely evaluation and management at the first signs of a potential infection. Fortunately, with greater access to diagnostic testing and appropriate antimicrobial therapy, the prognosis has improved over the years. Most significantly, it has been the recognition that early surgical intervention in appropriately selected patients also substantially improved the short- and long-term outcomes.

Endocarditis represents one of the few areas of medicine that require an aggressive and timely response by a multidisciplinary team. The spectrum of problems and presentation of patients require a rapid response to determine an effective care plan. Such plans must be open to reevaluation continuously as the clinical course can be difficult to predict. Good team communication cannot be overemphasized. As guidelines and protocols continue to evolve and assist in patient management, the variability in disease presentation requires each case to be individualized. While a single text on this topic would be overwhelming, the hope of this book is to highlight and provide modern insight into some of the current challenges and controversies that impact patient care directly.

Michael S. Firstenberg, MD FACC
Associate Professor of Surgery and Integrative Medicine
Northeast Ohio Medical Universities
Akron City Hospital - Summa Health System
Akron, Ohio, USA

Section 1

Introduction

Chapter 1

Introductory Chapter: Endocarditis - A Diagnostic and Therapeutic Challenge

Michael S. Firstenberg

Additional information is available at the end of the chapter

http://dx.doi.org/10.5772/66406

1. Introduction

Infective endocarditis (IE), reflecting infections of the heart—as manifested by vegetations on the valvular structures, abscess cavities of the myocardium, invasive fistula, or infections on intracardiac prosthetic devices—represents a significant problem that continues to challenge clinicians. The epidemiology of infections reflects not only the dark side of the progresses in medical therapy but also some of the social problems that plague modern society. The changing microbiology also reflects how this complex disease has also paralleled the advances in medicine. Diagnostic tools continue to evolve with not only improvements in imaging technologies but also our understandings on how to appropriately use them to better understand the overall clinical picture. In addition, the role of therapies—especially early surgical intervention—has been demonstrated to have a significant impact on the management and outcomes of infected patients. The goal of this text is to highlight some of the current concepts in the clinical characteristics, presentation, diagnosis, and management options.

2. Epidemiology

The incidence of infectious endocarditis, without a doubt, has increased significantly over the years. The reasons for this are multifactorial and reflect the growing number of patients who are at risk due to their comorbidities. The list of comorbidities is extensive and includes advancing age, chronic immunosuppression, end-stage renal failure, and those with pre-existing intracardiac pathology. Furthermore, as patients are living longer and longer with more complex comorbidities, medical teams are seeing the pathological consequences of some of the therapies that such patients require to prolong their lives. The dramatic increase in the use of cardiac support devices, such as pacemaker, defibrillators, intravascular monitoring devices, and left ventricular assist devices has presented unique and difficult challenges in management when patients are clinically dependent on them and then they become infected and may need to be removed. Clearly, endocarditis is one of those opportunistic problems that result from medical advances. However, without doubt, the largest populations of patients developing endocarditis are those with a history of intravenous drug abuse or those with a history of implanted cardiac devices [1, 2]. The undeniable worldwide epidemic of intravenous drug abuse has resulted in a dramatic increase in the incidence of younger patients presenting with polymicrobial invasive infections—often in the setting of overwhelming sepsis and difficult to manage social situations with established concerns of noncompliance. In this patient population, the primary cardiac infections might be the easiest of their presenting problems to manage long term. The other major patient population at significant risk is those with underlying cardiovascular pathologies requiring implantable support devices and lead system. In addition, the increasing long-term survival of patients with prosthetic heart valves, corrected congenital heart disease, and wider use of percutaneously implanted cardiac valves (i.e., TAVR) or repair devices (i.e., mitral clips) in high-risk surgical patients also place these patients at risk for device-related infection and the increasing incidence of endocarditis [3]. It is also becoming concerning, as discussed in this text, that infections in certain patient populations—such as those with end-stage renal disease requiring hemodialysis—are at substantial risk for endocarditis and life-threatening complications in ways that are only recently being appreciated and described in the literature. Nevertheless, guidelines for prophylactic antibiotics remain unclear in how "at risk" patients should be managed at the time of invasive procedures that might predispose to bacteremia and subsequent seeding of cardiac, native and prosthetic, structures [4–6]. To say that there is much controversy in this area is an understatement.

3. Microbiology

The microbiology of IE has also evolved over the years. The growing incidence of difficult-to-treat infections, methicillin-resistant Staphylococcus, polymicrobial infections with Gram-negative bacteria, primary or opportunistic fungi, and multidrug-resistant organisms has also increased the difficulties in managing this patient population—and is independently a predictor of worse outcomes and hence is often an indication for urgent surgery [7]. Advances in the ability of microbiology labs to better identify unusual organisms—including genetic material—have allowed for more accurately defining causative agents that otherwise would have been considered "culture negative." Furthermore, as more aggressive approaches to the diagnosis and management of sepsis have resulted in a more assertive approach to insuring appropriate and timely cultures, antibiotics, and a search of an infectious focus, there might be a more accurate and timely diagnosis of extensive bacterial infections [8], while it is unclear whether such an aggressive approach toward "septic" patients has changed the incidence of endocarditis or whether the significant increase in case presentations is more of a function of an overall awareness. Without doubt, as resistance patterns emerge within a community and a patient presents, for many reasons, with more unusual infectious, these patterns are also reflected in the microbiologic picture of endocarditis. In addition, the increase in immune modulating medications has also increased the incidence of fungal infections and very unusual pathogens [9]. Similarly, as patients with adult congenital heart disease and prosthetic material live longer, their overall risk of developing unusual infections that evolve into endocarditis also increases [10, 11].

In addition, as discussed in this text, there is a growing body of literature on concepts such as culture negative endocarditis and noninfectious endocarditis such as marantic or Libman-Sacks endocarditis [12].

4. Diagnosis

Positive blood cultures remain the *sine quo non* in the diagnosis of endocarditis—but the corollary is not always true as patients can present with significant valvular pathology and negative cultures. The Duke Criteria, discussed at length elsewhere and in this text, remain the cornerstones for the diagnosis of endocarditis [13]. Advances in imaging, much like advances in the microbiologic assessment, of patients has also contributed significantly to the diagnosis and management of infected patients [14]. While transthoracic and transesophageal imaging are still first-line diagnostic tests to evaluate potentially infected cardiac structures—and current guidelines help outline appropriateness criteria [2, 12]—there are growing indications and roles for alternative imaging modalities such as the computed tomography (CT), magnetic resonance imaging, and even 3D echocardiography [15]. As discussed in this text—advanced imaging modalities clearly have an expanding role in the diagnosis and management of patient with endocarditis. Early and frequent imaging can be extremely helpful in guiding and assessing the response to therapy.

5. Therapy

As well described and discussed at length in several chapters of this book, successful management of endocarditis requires a multidisciplinary approach. Clearly targeted and appropriate antibiotics are necessary. Prolonged courses of intravenous antibiotics are often prescribed, and fortunately, most patients can receive their therapies as an outpatient with close follow-up. While social and economic variables, not to mention restrictions by insurance companies and funding agencies, may limit options, fortunately from a medical standpoint, most patients will tolerate a prolonged course of antibiotics.

However, the critical decision-making regarding treatment for endocarditis is focused on appropriate interventional or surgical management. When associated with pacemaker lead systems or intracardiac devices, especially in the setting of large vegetations and resistant organisms or fungal infections, current guidelines advocate early and aggressive removal of all artificial material. Obviously, this can be quite challenging from not only a technical standpoint when the patient is quite sick but also how to support a patient that may be pacemaker-dependent in the setting of an infected pacemaker lead system. While many such devices can be removed percutaneously, there is often concern that large vegetations or lead systems that are firmly adherent to cardiac structures such as the tricuspid valve may require open heart surgery with direct removal [16]. Again, such cases illustrate the importance of a multidisciplinary team approach to not only the timing of interventions but also the specific procedures that may be required to remove the offending hardware.

The greater challenge is the timing of surgical intervention in patients who may require valve surgery—either repair or replacement—especially in the setting of associated other intracardiac pathology. Historical paradigms of prolonged courses of antibiotics and delayed surgical intervention, often after completion of a course of antibiotics, have been challenged recently as current European and American Society guidelines are tending to advocate early and aggressive surgical intervention. It was believed previously that early surgery and patients with active infections and vegetations were associated with a prohibitive risk for reinfection and postoperative complications from operating on septic patients. This was the rationale for delayed surgery after a prolonged course of antibiotics [17]. However, this approach was frequently criticized as selecting only those patients who survived complication free to complete their course of antibiotics, while potentially undertreating those patients who may have benefited from aggressive debridement and infection source control and who ultimately died of either overwhelming septic complications or catastrophic neurological events. A randomized trial of 37 patients with left-sided endocarditis, severe valvular disease, and large vegetations compared early surgical intervention with conventional medical therapies and potential delayed interval surgery and concluded that early surgery had a significant impact in reducing further embolic events and death [18]. Unfortunately, as a function of the nature of the disease combined with associated comorbidities, randomized trials dealing with surgical management of infected endocarditis can be very difficult. Current guidelines acknowledge this fact and base their recommendations on the growing body of literature that consists predominantly of small series and high-quality observational studies [19]. Nevertheless, the current guidelines suggest early surgical intervention in those patients who present with the following characteristics:

1. Valvular dysfunction resulting in signs or symptoms of acute heart failure.
2. Early surgery is recommended with those patients with fungal infections or highly resistant organisms.
3. Those patients who present with cardiovascular complications directly associated with their infections, including new heart block, aortic or root or annular abscess cavities, or penetrating infectious complications such as fistula, might benefit from early surgery.
4. Surgery is indicated in the setting of persistent bacteremia or fever greater than 5–7 days in the absence of another identifiable primary source in the setting of appropriate targeted antibiotic therapy.

5. Enlarging vegetations despite appropriate antibiotic therapy or evidence of recurrent embolic complications.

6. Vegetations that are mobile and greater than 1 cm and/or with evidence of severe valve regurgitation.

7. Mobile vegetations that are greater than 1 cm especially in the setting of other relative indications for surgery and when involving the anterior leaflet of the mitral valve.

Similar recommendations are used to guide therapy in patients with prosthetic valve endocarditis [20]. However, it must be considered that overall, prosthetic valve endocarditis can be very difficult to successfully manage medically.

A growing challenge is the population presenting with right-sided endocarditis especially in the setting of poly-microbial or resistant organisms from intravenous drug abuse. Again, historically because of the concerns of recurrent infections or relapse, there was reluctance to intervene early, and many of these patients were treated medically. However, there is growing evidence that tricuspid valve surgery should be considered in those patients with worsening right heart failure from tricuspid regurgitation, failure of medical therapy, difficult to treat organisms, vegetations greater than 2 cm, and worsening pulmonary complications from presumed septic pulmonary emboli. Obviously, the challenge is not only patient selection but also surgical timing—again emphasizing the importance of a multidisciplinary team to sort out the clinical issues [21]. Historical management of tricuspid pathology was often "vegectomy" or "valvectomy" [22]. While there were some survivors of such therapy, without doubt, the developing of acute and chronic right heart failure and the consequences of it—such as hepatic congestion and failure—limit the practical application of such approaches [23]. Rarely is right-side infections managed with procedures that result in severe regurgitation—a pathophysiology that is often the initial indication for intervention.

Nevertheless, the growing consensus is that patients with severe valvular infections especially in the setting of failure of appropriate medical therapy, worsening vegetations, systemic complications, and especially worsening heart failure should be promptly evaluated and considered for early, if not urgent, surgical intervention. Obviously, the risks and benefits of surgery in a septic patient with associated comorbidities must be evaluated on a case-by-case basis and take into consideration vocal experiences and resources.

6. Social implications

Without doubt, the greatest challenges in dealing with patients with endocarditis are the growing population of patients presenting with a history of intravenous drug abuse—especially heroin. Recent data suggest a twofold increase in the number of active users of heroin between 2006 and 2013 [24]. The growing epidemic of drug abuse, worldwide, cannot be ignored nor denied. Endocarditis in the setting of IV drug abuse is particularly difficult to manage, while the etiology is often the use of infected needles or contamination of the drugs being directly injected into the vascular system. Patients who present with infections also have other acquired comorbidities associated with their substance abuse that challenge their management and long-term prognosis. Hepatitis B and C as well as human immunodeficiency virus are often encountered in this patient population [25]. Chronic pain syndromes as well as their underlying drug addiction and associated personality and psychological disorders not only makes this population difficult to manage in the hospital setting but also raises the concern of long-term compliance with medical therapies. While there might be a general reluctance, for example, to use mechanical valves in younger patients, concerns about compliance with anticoagulation often leaves little choice. This is particularly true when patients present with a history of hepatitis and their long-term liver function (critical for clotting factors and Coumadin management) is unpredictable. Without doubt, this population is at risk for recurrent problems secondary to their substance abuse history. A recent study by Kim and colleagues illustrate the scope of this problem. Between 2002 and 2014, there was a twofold increase in the number of patients requiring surgery for infected endocarditis at their institution space (14.8% in 2002–26% in 2012). Of the 436 patients studied, over a mean follow-up of 29 months adverse events occurred in 20% including 10% developing re-infections—often as a function of continued substance abuse. While their findings demonstrated a lower operative mortality in patients with drug abuse predominately as a function of their age, propensity score analysis indicated that IV drug abuse was associated with an almost fourfold increase in valve-related complications and a 6.2-fold increase in reinfection. Because of the concerns of noncompliance, relapse of drug abuse, and poor socioeconomic status of many of these patients, surgical intervention in the setting of long-standing drug abuse is often viewed as intervening on an end-stage, often inherently fatal, disease. Some clinicians viewed attempts at curing these patients of their infections and substance abuse as being futile. In fact, while often discussed but rarely written, most programs will refuse surgical re-intervention except for extenuating circumstances in those patients who continue to demonstrate ongoing drug abuse who subsequently developed recurrent prosthetic valve infections. Prior to refusing potentially lifesaving, but high-risk, surgery in such patients or referral to palliative care, an open and honest discussion with an Institutional Ethics Team might be indicated.

Because of the cost of therapy that often includes prolonged hospitalizations, extensive diagnostic evaluations, complex surgery, or multiple surgical interventions, and often a prolonged recovery that can also be challenged by baseline comorbidities, disease complications, and access to potentially limited resources, the growing epidemic of endocarditis is clearly a problem. This is all in the background of whether the social programs that reduce the risk of infections, such as prophylactic antibiotics prior to dental procedures, are cost effective or even reduce the risk of infections at all [26, 27]

7. Conclusion

As technology has improved over the years, so has the ability to detect and guide the management of patients with infections. This has also paralleled the significant increase in the incidence of such infections as patients get older, develop more comorbidities (especially from lifestyle choices), have more implanted devices that can potentially get infected, and have more procedures that might infect cardiac structures (both native and prosthetic). Endocarditis remains a formidable problem—both in terms of diagnosis and management. Risks are high and, without doubt, a team approach is crucial to the successful management of these patients (**Figure 1**) [28, 29].

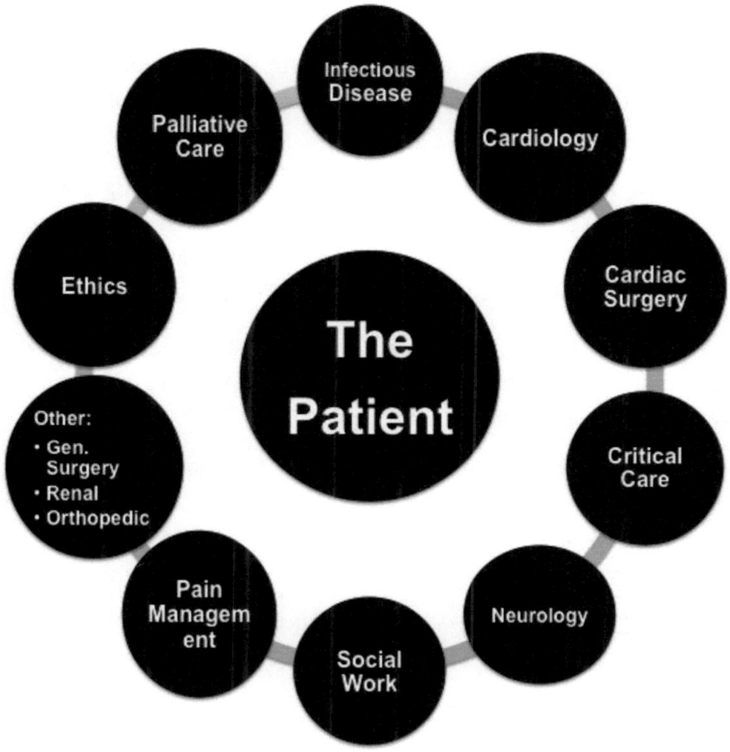

Figure 1. Components of an "Endocarditis Heart Team"—all focused on the patient.

While the goal of this text is not to be an all-inclusive reference on this topic—the hope is that it will provide a current update on some of the key topics that reflect the multiple, evolving, and difficult challenges in the assessment and therapies available for such a devastating problem.

Author details

Michael S. Firstenberg

Address all correspondence to: msfirst@gmail.com

Department of Surgery (Cardiothoracic), Northeast Ohio Medical University, Akron City Hospital—Summa Health System, Akron, Ohio, USA

References

[1] Sousa, C., Botelho, C., Rodrigues, D., Azeredo, J. and Oliveira, R., 2012. Infective endocarditis in intravenous drug abusers: an update. *European Journal of Clinical Microbiology & Infectious Diseases*, 31(11), pp. 2905–2910.

[2] Habib, G., Lancellotti, P., Antunes, M.J., Bongiorni, M.G., Casalta, J.P., Del Zotti, F., Dulgheru, R., El Khoury, G., Erba, P.A., Iung, B. and Miro, J.M., 2015. 2015 ESC Guidelines for the management of infective endocarditis. *European Heart Journal*, p. ehv319.

[3] Latib, A., Naim, C., De Bonis, M., Sinning, J.M., Maisano, F., Barbanti, M., Parolari, A., Lorusso, R., Testa, L., Dato, G.M.A. and Miceli, A., 2014. TAVR-associated prosthetic valve infective endocarditis: results of a large, multicenter registry. *Journal of the American College of Cardiology*, 64(20), pp. 2176–2178.

[4] Thornhill, M.H., Dayer, M.J., Jones, S., Prendergast, B., Baddour, L.M. and Lockhart, P.B., 2016. The effect of antibiotic prophylaxis guidelines on incidence of infective endocarditis. *Canadian Journal of Cardiology*.

[5] Patanè, S., 2014. Is there a need for bacterial endocarditis prophylaxis in patients undergoing gastrointestinal endoscopy? *Journal of Cardiovascular Translational Research*, 7(3), pp. 372–374.

[6] Dayer, M.J., Jones, S., Prendergast, B., Baddour, L.M., Lockhart, P.B. and Thornhill, M.H., 2015. Incidence of infective endocarditis in England, 2000–13: a secular trend, interrupted time-series analysis. *The Lancet*, 385(9974), pp. 1219–1228.

[7] Slipczuk, L., Codolosa, N.J., Carlos, D., Romero-Corral, A., Pressman, G.S. and Figueredo, V.M., 2012. Systematic review and meta-analysis of infective endocarditis microbiology over 5 decades. *Circulation*, 126(Suppl 21), pp. A15138–A15138.

[8] Dellinger, R.P., Levy, M.M., Rhodes, A., Annane, D., Gerlach, H., Opal, S.M., Sevransky, J.E., Sprung, C.L., Douglas, I.S., Jaeschke, R. and Osborn, T.M., 2013. Surviving Sepsis Campaign: international guidelines for management of severe sepsis and septic shock, 2012. *Intensive Care Medicine*, 39(2), pp. 165–228.

[9] Tacke, D., Koehler, P. and Cornely, O.A., 2013. Fungal endocarditis. *Current Opinion in Infectious Diseases*, 26(6), pp. 501–507.

[10] Abandeh, F.I., Bazan, J.A., Davis, J.A., Zaidi, A.N., Daniels, C.J. and Firstenberg, M.S., 2012. Bartonella henselae prosthetic valve endocarditis in an adult patient with congenital heart disease: favorable outcome after combined medical and surgical management. *Journal of Cardiac Surgery*, 27(4), pp. 449–452.

[11] Pfahl, K.W., Orsinelli, D.A., Raman, S. and Firstenberg, M., 2013. The diagnosis and treatment of a mycotic coronary artery aneurysm: a case report. *Echocardiography*, 30(10), pp. E304–E306.

[12] Liu J, Frishman W. Nonbacterial thrombotic endocarditis-pathogenesis, diagnosis and management. *Cardiology in Review*. April 26, 2016 .

[13] Baddour, L.M., Wilson, W.R., Bayer, A.S., Fowler, V.G., Tleyjeh, I.M., Rybak, M.J., Barsic, B., Lockhart, P.B., Gewitz, M.H., Levison, M.E. and Bolger, A.F., 2015. Infective endocarditis in adults: diagnosis, antimicrobial therapy, and management of complications a scientific statement for healthcare professionals from the American Heart Association. *Circulation*, 132(15), pp. 1435–1486.

[14] Bruun, N.E., Habib, G., Thuny, F. and Sogaard, P., 2014. Cardiac imaging in infectious endocarditis. *European Heart Journal*, 35(10), pp.624–632.

[15] Habets, J., Tanis, W., Reitsma, J.B., van den Brink, R.B., Willem, P.T.M., Chamuleau, S.A. and Budde, R.P., 2015. Are novel non-invasive imaging techniques needed in patients with suspected prosthetic heart valve endocarditis? A systematic review and meta-analysis. *European Radiology*, 25(7), pp. 2125–2133.

[16] Koutentakis, M., Siminelakis, S., Korantzopoulos, P., Petrou, A., Priavali, E., Mpakas, A., Gesouli, E., Apostolakis, E., Tsakiridis, K., Zarogoulidis, P. and Katsikogiannis, N., 2014. Surgical management of cardiac implantable electronic device infections. *Journal of Thoracic Disease*, 6(1), pp.S173–S179.

[17] Aranki, S.F., Santini, F., Adams, D.H., Rizzo, R.J., Couper, G.S., Kinchla, N.M., Gildea, J.S., Collins Jr, J.J. and Cohn, L.H., 1994. Aortic valve endocarditis. Determinants of early survival and late morbidity. *Circulation*, 90(5 Pt 2), pp. II175–II182.

[18] Kang, D.H., Kim, Y.J., Kim, S.H., Sun, B.J., Kim, D.H., Yun, S.C., Song, J.M., Choo, S.J., Chung, C.H., Song, J.K. and Lee, J.W., 2012. Early surgery versus conventional treatment for infective endocarditis. *New England Journal of Medicine*, 366(26), pp. 2466–2473.

[19] Erbel, R.A., 2014. The New strategy in infective endocarditis: early surgery based on early diagnosis: are we too late, when early surgery is best? *Circulation*, pp. CIRCULATIONAHA–114.

[20] Perrotta, S., Jeppsson, A., Fröjd, V. and Svensson, G., 2016. Surgical treatment of aortic prosthetic valve endocarditis: a 20-year single-center experience. *The Annals of Thoracic Surgery*, 101(4), pp. 1426–1432.

[21] Yong, M.S., Coffey, S., Prendergast, B.D., Marasco, S.F., Zimmet, A.D., McGiffin, D.C. and Saxena, P., 2016. Surgical management of tricuspid valve endocarditis in the current era: a review. *International Journal of Cardiology*, 202, pp. 44–48.

[22] Hughes CF, Noble N., 1988. Vegetectomy: an alternative surgical treatment for infective endocarditis of the atrioventricular valves in drug addicts. *Journal of Thoracic Cardiovascular Surgery*, 95, pp. 857–861

[23] Dawood, M.Y., Cheema, F.H., Ghoreishi, M., Foster, N.W., Villanueva, R.M., Salenger, R., Griffith, B.P. and Gammie, J.S., 2015. Contemporary outcomes of operations for tricuspid valve infective endocarditis. *The Annals of Thoracic Surgery*, 99(2), pp. 539–546.

[24] Wurcel, A.G., Anderson, J.E., Chui, K.K., Skinner, S., Knox, T.A., Snydman, D.R. and Stopka, T.J., 2016, May. Increasing infectious endocarditis admissions among young people who inject drugs. In: *Open Forum Infectious Diseases* (Vol. 3, No. 3, p. 157). Oxford University Press.

[25] Gundelly, P., Burgess, D.S., Boulay, J., Caldwell, G. and Thornton, A., 2014, December. 921 Prevalence of hepatitis C infection and epidemiology of infective endocarditis in intravenous drug users in central Kentucky. In *Open Forum Infectious Diseases* (Vol. 1, No. Suppl 1, pp. S266–S266). Oxford University Press.

[26] Wray, D., Ruiz, F., Richey, R. and Stokes, T. 2008. Prophylaxis against infective endocarditis for dental procedures–summary of the NICE guideline. *British Dental Journal,* 204(10), pp. 555–557.

[27] Sunder, S., Grammatico-Guillon, L., Baron, S., Gaborit, C., Bernard-Brunet, A., Garot, D., Legras, A., Prazuck, T., Dibon, O., Boulain, T. and Tabone, X., 2015. Clinical and economic outcomes of infective endocarditis. *Infectious Diseases,* 47(2), pp. 80–87.

[28] Chambers, J., Sandoe, J., Ray, S., Prendergast, B., Taggart, D., Westaby, S., Arden, C., Grothier, L., Wilson, J., Campbell, B. and Gohlke-Bärwolf, C., 2014. The infective endocarditis team: recommendations from an international working group. *Heart,* 100(7), pp. 524–527.

[29] Chirillo, F., Scotton, P., Rocco, F., Rigoli, R., Polesel, E. and Olivari, Z., 2013. Management of patients with infective endocarditis by a multidisciplinary team approach: an operative protocol. *Journal of Cardiovascular Medicine,* 14(9), pp. 659–668.

Section 2

Prevention and Epidemiology

Chapter 2

Antibiotic Prophylactic Regimens for Infective Endocarditis in Patients Undergoing Dental Procedures

Miguel Castro, Javier Álvarez, Javier F. Feijoo, Marcio Diniz, Lucía García-Caballero, Pedro Diz and Jacobo Limeres

Additional information is available at the end of the chapter

http://dx.doi.org/10.5772/65255

Abstract

Up to date causal relationship has been demonstrated between dental manipulations and the onset of infective endocarditis (IE). However, since 1955, numerous expert committees have proposed antibiotic prophylaxis (AP) to prevent bacteraemia of oral origin. Controversy regarding the efficacy of AP prior to the dental procedures has intensified in recent years because of the lack of conclusive evidence on its efficacy for the prevention of IE and on its cost-effectiveness, as well as the possibility of allergic reactions and the emergence of antibiotic resistance. Accordingly, AP is now maintained exclusively for patients at highest risk and who require the manipulation of the gingival or periapical regions of the teeth or perforation of the oral mucosa. In the context of a restrictive policy, the National Institute for Health and Clinical Excellence (NICE) of the United Kingdom published a new guideline in 2008 stating that "AP against IE is not recommended for persons undergoing dental procedures", regardless of risk status and of the nature of the procedure to be performed. The NICE guideline has generated further controversy, and expert committees in other countries continue to publish prophylactic regimens for the prevention of IE secondary to dental procedures. In this chapter, we discuss the principal guidelines currently applicable in Europe, the USA and Australia, and we draw particular attention to the need for randomised clinical trials.

Keywords: infective endocarditis, bacteraemia, dental procedures, dentistry, antibiotic prophylaxis

1. Historical perspectives

In 1955, the American Heart Association (AHA) was the first medical society to establish the need for a prophylactic antibiotic regimen to prevent infective endocarditis (IE) in at-risk patients undergoing various surgical procedures, including tooth extractions and other dental manipulations that affect the gum.

In the pre-antibiotic era, reports based on clinical observations described cases of IE of streptococcal aetiology in which there was a history of professional dental manipulation. This suggested the possibility that "transient bacteraemia during dental procedures may lead to subacute endocarditis in subjects with abnormal heart valves" [1].

The 1955 AHA Committee on the Prevention of Rheumatic Fever and Bacterial Endocarditis concluded that patients undergoing dental procedures must be protected by high concentrations of antibiotic present in the blood at the time of the procedure. Penicillin administered parenterally was preferred, although oral penicillin V was introduced as second choice. In cases of sensitivity to penicillin, other antibiotics such erythromycin or tetracycline were recommended [2].

Since that time, the scientific community has universally accepted the need for antibiotic prophylaxis in patients susceptible to developing IE. Experimental models developed in the 1970s provided evidence of the efficacy of prophylaxis in animals and demonstrated the ability of antibiotics to prevent *Streptococcus sanguinis* endocarditis [3]. However, the different antibiotic regimens to prevent IE in dental patients were developed based on empirical criteria.

In 1982, the British Society for Antimicrobial Chemotherapy included amoxicillin in the prophylactic antibiotic regimen against IE [4]. Amoxicillin has a broad antibacterial spectrum and a more favourable pharmacokinetic profile than penicillin V for oral administration; this has made it the drug of choice in all current guidelines on the use of antibiotics to prevent IE.

The main inclusion criteria for the prophylactic regimens established by the first committees were the rheumatic heart disease and congenital malformations, but fundamental changes have been introduced since that time regarding "patients considered to be at risk of IE". The campaigns for the prevention of rheumatic fever, the increase in the prevalence of intravenous drug abuse and the growth in cardiovascular interventions have transformed the microbiological patterns of IE, with a relative decrease in the incidence of streptococcal endocarditis and a significant increase in endocarditis due to staphylococci and other less common organisms.

These changes make it difficult to draw reliable epidemiological conclusions on the efficacy of antibiotics for the prevention of IE. In general, the majority of studies indicate that, despite the universal implantation of antibiotic prophylaxis prior to the dental treatment, no global reduction in the prevalence of IE has been achieved [5].

This has been one of the main arguments put forward by the British health authorities to revoke the indications for antibiotic prophylaxis in patients undergoing dental, digestive tract or genitourinary interventions. A few years ago, the National Institute for Health and Clinical

Excellence (NICE) in the United Kingdom published a proposal that surprised the scientific community by considering that "antibiotic prophylaxis for IE was not recommended for persons undergoing dental treatment". This recommendation was even applicable to "high-risk patients, independently of the type of dental procedure they were to undergo" [6].

This scepticism of the British health authorities to the prophylactic efficacy of antibiotics in IE is not shared by other scientific societies, which continue to include antibiotic cover for dental procedures in patients at risk of developing IE.

Epidemiological observations and statistical analyses made after the cessation of prophylaxis in the United Kingdom suggest the need for antibiotic cover in patients at maximum risk of IE of poor prognosis. In this setting, current guidelines maintain the need for prevention for patients considered to be at high risk of developing IE, such as individuals with prosthetic heart valves, the presence of certain congenital cardiopathies and patients who have had a previous episode of IE.

2. Impact of the nice recommendations

In the controversial document published in 2008, NICE brought about the complete cessation of antibiotic prophylaxis for all patients at risk of IE undergoing dental interventions [6]. The main premises on which the British experts based this decision was the quantifiable risk of antibiotic administration to the individual patient, the potential appearance of unnecessary antimicrobial resistance and the economic analysis of the cost-effectiveness of prophylaxis.

The recommendation was based on the limited available evidence on antibiotic prophylaxis as an effective method to reduce the incidence of IE when given before an interventional procedure. Furthermore, the existence of transient bacteraemia during activities of daily living, such as toothbrushing or chewing, diminishes the significance of dental procedures as a cause of IE, making antibiotic prophylaxis virtually ineffective for preventing the disease.

Consequently, NICE did not recommend antibiotic prophylaxis against IE in persons undergoing dental procedures or digestive, respiratory or genitourinary tract interventions, except for manipulations at an infected non-dental site.

The expert committees across the rest of the world, including the AHA and the European Society of Cardiology (ESC), have continued to recommend antibiotic prophylaxis in high-risk individuals, and these protocols are followed by most cardiologists and cardiac surgeons.

The first studies on the epidemiological repercussions of the implementation of the NICE guideline showed a substantial reduction in the prescription of antibiotics in its area of influence and the data gathered showed no significant changes in the general upward trend in cases of IE [7].

In 2013, a case of IE was reported in which aetiological analysis suggested a very strong association with a previous dental intervention performed without antibiotic cover. The affected patient had a metallic aortic valve and developed a fatal episode of *S. sanguinis* endocarditis 10 days after undergoing a dental procedure without antibiotic prophylaxis, following the NICE recommendations. The dental history of the patient showed that he had received antibiotic prophylaxis during dental sessions over the previous 10 years with no adverse outcomes [8].

The most recent epidemiological studies have identified a significant increase in the incidence of IE after implementation of the NICE guideline. A retrospective study was performed in England to investigate the effect of antibiotic prophylaxis versus no prophylaxis on the incidence of IE [9]. The data collected and the subsequent analysis suggested that after March 2008—the year of publication of the NICE guideline—the number of cases of IE increased significantly above the expected historical trend.

According to some experts, these data are mainly observational and do not prove that the lower level of antibiotic prophylaxis was the cause of the increase in IE. However, no other satisfactory explanation for this increase in the incidence of IE has yet been put forward [10].

Despite this, NICE has reviewed all evidence relating to the effectiveness of IE prophylaxis as a precaution but, at present, they have found no need to change any of the existing 2008 guideline. They have, however, made an additional research recommendations on antibiotic prophylaxis against IE as summarised in **Table 1**.

Field of research	Importance
1. National register of infective endocarditis	To provide a cohort of patients able to generate sufficient evidence from well-conducted national studies
2. Cardiac conditions and infective endocarditis	To use a population-based cohort study design to allow direct comparison between acquired heart valve disease and structural congenital heart disease to estimate relative and absolute IE risk
3. Interventional procedures and infective endocarditis	To determine the frequency and intensity of bacteraemia caused by non-oral daily activities
4. Antibiotic prophylaxis against infective endocarditis	A randomised controlled trial with long-term follow-up comparing antibiotic prophylaxis with no antibiotic prophylaxis in adults and children with underlying structural heart defects undergoing interventional procedures

Note: https://nice.org.uk/guidance/CG64/chapter/Recommendations-for-research#4-antibiotic-prophylaxis-against-infective-endocarditis

Table 1. NICE recommendations for research. Antimicrobial prophylaxis against infective endocarditis in adults and children undergoing interventional procedures (updated in 2015).

3. Current antibiotic protocols

Antibiotic prophylaxis protocols against IE have undergone relevant changes in recent years. There is no doubt that the categorical 2008 NICE recommendations and their implementation in their area of influence constitute an event with significant epidemiological repercussions

http://dx.doi.org/10.5772/65255

that will serve to evaluate the efficacy of antibiotic prophylaxis for the prevention of IE. The scientific societies responsible for this question continue detailed follow-up in order to incorporate their conclusions as relevant data arise.

Among the different prophylaxis guidelines proposed by expert committees around the world, those that represent their corresponding geographical areas stand out for their scientific relevance. In the USA, the AHA has been pioneer in the introduction of antibiotic prophylaxis against IE; its most recent guideline was published in 2007 [11]. In Australia, the Infective Endocarditis Prophylaxis Expert Group (AIEPEG) published a guideline in 2008 that has been supported by the principal health associations in its area of influence [12]. In Europe, the ESC published the 2015 review of its protocols in the European Heart Journal, stating the official position of that scientific society on this subject [13]. These three guidelines coincide on two major points:

- All propose amoxicillin as the antibiotic of choice.
- All propose clindamycin as the alternative antibiotic of choice to amoxicillin.

3.1. Amoxicillin as the antibiotic of choice for prophylaxis

The standard regimens of the three guidelines mentioned above recommend the oral administration of 2 g of amoxicillin between 30 and 60 min before a dental procedure in adults. In the case of children, the recommended dose is 50 mg/kg body weight. When oral administration is not possible, amoxicillin can be administered intramuscularly or intravenously at the same dose.

Amoxicillin was introduced into the IE prophylaxis protocols in 1982 [4] and since that time it has become the drug of choice in the prophylactic guidelines internationally. From a pharmacological point of view, amoxicillin has optimal characteristics due to its rapid absorption after administration by mouth, achieving maximum plasma concentrations within 1–2 h after ingestion, and therapeutic levels are maintained for a minimum of 6 h. Amoxicillin is highly active against streptococci and also covers anaerobes and gram-negative bacteria. It is thus effective against the majority of microorganisms present in bacteraemia of oral origin. However, it is considered that between 5 and 35% of the microorganisms detected in blood cultures from patients undergoing dental treatment can be resistant to the antibiotic. This finding, together with the increased prevalence of IE caused by penicillin-resistant staphylococci and other unusual microorganisms, could justify the introduction of antibiotics other than amoxicillin into standard prophylaxis protocols in the future in order to improve the antimicrobial spectrum in certain circumstances.

3.2. Alternative drugs to amoxicillin

The three guidelines incorporate cephalosporins for parenteral administration as an alternative to amoxicillin. The cephalosporins are also recommended in patients with penicillin allergy, though this proposal is accompanied by a warning that the use of cephalosporins is contraindicated in individuals with a history of anaphylaxis.

About 10% of patients attending dental consultations are allergic to penicillin and its derivatives, although a large majority of these reported allergic reactions are no more than minor side-effects or late hypersensitivity reactions presenting as pruritus or rash, but not IgE-mediated. Urticaria (hives) is IgE-mediated; it only accounts for 10% of all exanthematous drug reactions, but may be interpreted as a clinical sign of immediate hypersensitivity that could progress to an episode of acute (fulminant) anaphylaxis.

The main antigenic determinant of the anaphylactic reaction to penicillins is the β-lactam ring, a part of the molecule that is essential for its bactericidal activity and that also forms part of the chemical structure of the cephalosporins and clavulanates (clavulanic acid), among others. Drug-related anaphylaxis is a life-threatening medical emergency and, as a result, the administration of β-lactam drugs is contraindicated in patients who give a history of penicillin allergy until such time as allergy testing establishes the true risk of anaphylaxis in each individual case [14].

The three main guidelines coincide on the oral or intravenous administration of 600 mg of clindamycin as the antibiotic of choice in patients allergic to penicillins (**Table 2**). Clindamycin has intrinsic in vitro activity against streptococci, staphylococci and anaerobes, it rarely causes allergic reactions and it has a low incidence of side-effects, making it an ideal alternative antibiotic based on its antimicrobial spectrum and biosafety. However, some authors have demonstrated that it is ineffective in preventing bacteraemia following dental procedures [15].

Australia (AIEPEG)	Europe (ESC)	USA (AHA)
Clindamycin	Clindamycin	Clindamycin
Lincomycin		Azithromycin
Vancomycin		Clarithromycin
Teicoplanin		

Abbreviations: AIEPEG, Australian Infective Endocarditis Prophylaxis Expert Group; ESC, European Society of Cardiology; AHA, American Heart Association.

Table 2. Alternative antibiotics for prophylaxis against infective endocarditis in patients allergic to penicillins and their derivatives.

The 2007 AHA guideline describes in great detail specific situations that could require changes to the application of the prophylactic regimens in clinical practice. For example, intramuscular injections should be avoided in patients receiving anticoagulants. In patients attending the dental clinic whilst on treatment with penicillins for other causes, it is preferable to delay dental therapy for at least 10 days; it is accepted that viridans group streptococci in the oral cavity of patients on long-term antibiotic therapy could be relatively resistant to penicillin or amoxicillin, and the cessation of antibiotic therapy allows the usual oral flora to be re-established. When the dental intervention cannot be postponed, the health professional should select a different class of antibiotic rather than increase the dose of the current antibiotic; options include clindamycin, azithromycin and clarithromycin, though only for patients with the highest-risk cardiac conditions [11].

Azithromycin and clarithromycin are macrolides with similar activity to erythromycin on the oral streptococci, but they show better gastrointestinal tolerance and a more favourable pharmacokinetic profile. Erythromycin is unstable under acidic gastric conditions, shows poor absorption and has a limited spectrum of activity. Azithromycin, on the other hand, causes fewer gastrointestinal side-effects, rapidly reaches high tissue concentrations and displays a better antibacterial spectrum, making it a good candidate for IE prophylaxis [16].

The Australian guideline includes a parenteral regimen of lincomycin, vancomycin or teicoplanin for patients with penicillin hypersensitivity and for those on long-term penicillin therapy or who have taken penicillin or related β-lactam antibiotics more than once in the previous month [12].

Finally, the ESC guideline is the most restrictive, recommending clindamycin as the only alternative antibiotic. In contrast to the proposal of the Australian expert committee, the European guideline states that the glycopeptides, such as vancomycin and teicoplanin, are not recommended because their efficacy has not been fully demonstrated and there is a potential for the induction of resistance [13].

4. At-risk patients

In its conclusions, the 2007 AHA guideline states that IE prophylaxis for dental procedures is a reasonable practice only for patients with underlying heart conditions associated with the highest risk of an adverse outcome [11]. New pathophysiological concepts and risk-benefit analyses justify the current tendency of the scientific community towards more limited indications for antibiotic prophylaxis in IE (**Table 3**).

1.	Bacteraemia occurs repeatedly and frequently during routine daily activities such as toothbrushing, flossing or chewing, and even more frequently in patients with poor dental health.
2.	Most case-control studies did not report an association between invasive dental procedures and the occurrence of infective endocarditis.
3.	The estimated risk of infective endocarditis following dental procedures is very low.
4.	Although antibiotic administration carries a small risk of anaphylaxis, it may become significant in the event of widespread use.
5.	Widespread use of antibiotics may result in the emergence of resistant microorganisms.
6.	Although efficacy of antibiotic prophylaxis on bacteraemia and the occurrence of infective endocarditis has been proven in animal models, the effect on bacteraemia in humans is controversial.
7.	No prospective randomised controlled trial has investigated the efficacy of antibiotic prophylaxis on the occurrence of infective endocarditis.

Table 3. Arguments for the restriction of the indication for prophylaxis against infective endocarditis [13].

Epidemiological evidence also supports this restrictive policy, as the incidence of IE and its associated mortality have not varied in recent decades despite the use of antibiotic prophylaxis. At the present time, we are seeing an increase in the number of cases of IE due to *Staphylococcus aureus* and of unknown aetiology and a fall in the incidence of cases of IE of streptococcal aetiology [17]. This has occurred despite the evident, considerable increase in the number of dental interventions and in the ratio of dentists to population in recent years.

In this context and awaiting relevant new data, NICE in the UK continues its recommendation to universally cease antibiotic prophylaxis for medical interventions, although the majority of cardiologists and cardiac surgeons consider antibiotic prophylaxis necessary for patients at highest risk of adverse outcomes from endocarditis [9].

- Isolated secundum atrial septal defect.
- Surgical repair of atrial septal defect, ventricular septal defect, or patent ductus arteriosus (without residua beyond 6 months).
- Previous coronary artery bypass graft surgery.
- Mitral valve prolapse without valvar regurgitation.
- Physiologic, functional or innocent heart murmurs.
- Previous Kawasaki disease without valvar dysfunction.
- Previous rheumatic fever without valvar dysfunction.
- Cardiac pacemakers (intravascular and epicardial) and implanted defibrillators.

Table 4. Patients in whom prophylaxis against infective endocarditis is not recommended [18].

The 1997 AHA guideline was the first to stratify cardiac conditions into high, moderate and low risk for IE [18]. AHA experts stated that the risk of suffering IE assumed by low-risk patients undergoing dental treatment could be considered negligible, no higher than in the general population, and, as a result, they recommended abolishing antibiotic prophylaxis for routine dental treatment in these patients. This 1997 recommendation was particularly helpful in clinical practice because heart murmurs, pacemakers and minor congenital defects were frequently reported by dental patients in their medical records. The establishment of a restrictive position on the part of the health authorities regarding antibiotic prophylaxis created a framework of medico-legal protection in dental practice. The 1997 AHA guideline thus provided dentists with a certain capacity to evaluate the prescription of prophylaxis in patients with a history of cardiac disease and moderate their natural tendency to prescribe universal antibiotic cover derived from a fear of missing one of the numerous indications (**Table 4**). This conceptual change was further strengthened 10 years later when the 2007 AHA committee eliminated antibiotic prophylaxis for patients considered to be in the moderate risk category in the 1997 guideline (**Table 5**), on the basis that *"previously published AHA guidelines for the prevention of IE contained ambiguities and inconsistencies and were often based on minimal published data or expert opinion, they were subject to conflicting interpretations among patients, healthcare providers, and the legal system about patient eligibility for prophylaxis and whether there was strict adherence by healthcare providers to AHA recommendations for prophylaxis"* [11].

The current result of this policy limiting the indications for antibiotic prophylaxis to the highest risk cardiac conditions is stated even more restrictively in the 2015 ESC guideline (**Table 6**). In their recommendation, the ESC excludes prophylaxis even in heart transplant recipients who develop heart valve disease; this is considered a true high-risk condition in the AHA and Australian guidelines. The Australian recommendations also include rheumatic heart disease in indigenous Australians, a population in which unusually high prevalence and mortality related to this disease have been detected [19].

- Congenital cardiac conditions
  - ✓ Ductus arteriosus
  - ✓ Ventricular septal defect
  - ✓ Ostium primum atrial septal defect
  - ✓ Coarctation of the aorta
  - ✓ Bicuspid aortic valve
- Acquired valve dysfunction
  - ✓ Rheumatic
  - ✓ Collagen vascular disease
  - ✓ Others
- Hypertrophic cardiomyopathy
- Mitral valve prolapse with valve regurgitation and/or thickened leaflets

Table 5. Cardiac conditions that carry a moderate risk of infective endocarditis [18].

Finally, dental surgeons show a degree of concern over the need for prophylaxis when performing dental procedures on patients with implanted cardiac devices such as pacemakers, stents and implantable defibrillators. In 2007, Lockhart et al. published an interesting literature review on this subject, revealing widely differing opinions, a situation that usually leads dentists to contact physicians for advice on management. Interestingly, most physicians, surgeons and medical specialists want their patients to receive antibiotic prophylaxis for all invasive dental procedures to prevent distant site infection of organs, tissues or prosthetic materials, and a number of them do so for medico-legal rather than scientific reasons. The majority of the literature sources agree that there is no indication for prophylaxis in patients with cardiac devices. Bacterial seeding of a graft site via a haematogenous route is an uncommon event and most of infections occurring in the first 2 months are due to *Staphylococcus* spp. and non-oral bacteria, probably as result of the manoeuvres of graft placement [20].

Based on these premises, it could be stated that patients with implantable cardiac devices may be cautiously covered with antibiotic prophylaxis exclusively during the early post-implantation period, though this is mainly for medico-legal reasons. Considering the current IE prophylaxis guidelines, there is no reason for antibiotic use during routine dental treatment in patients with implantable cardiac devices, unless individual cases present concomitant diseases that could justify such a decision.

1. Patients with any prosthetic valve, including a transcatheter valve, or those in whom any prosthetic material was used for cardiac valve repair.
2. Patients with a previous episode of infective endocarditis.
3. Patients with congenital heart disease (CHD):
    a. Any type of cyanotic CHD.
    b. Any type of CHD repaired with a prosthetic material, whether placed surgically or by percutaneous techniques, up to 6 months after the procedure or lifelong if residual shunt or valvular regurgitation remains.

Table 6. Cardiac conditions associated with the highest risk of adverse outcomes of endocarditis according to the European Society of Cardiology guideline [13].

5. Risk-related dental procedures

In 1935, Okell and Elliott detected positive blood cultures in more than half of patients undergoing dental manipulations, with a particularly high prevalence among those with deficient oral health. Since that time, the relationship between bacteraemia of oral origin and dental interventions constituted proof that endocardial infection could be precipitated by oral streptococci mobilised during dental manipulation [21].

Transient bacteraemia has been widely documented as a common finding during dental procedures, associated particularly with the manipulation of teeth and periodontal tissues. Non-surgical tooth extraction is the dental procedure that most frequently provokes bacteraemia of oral origin, with a detection rate of positive blood cultures of 58–100% (**Figure 1**).

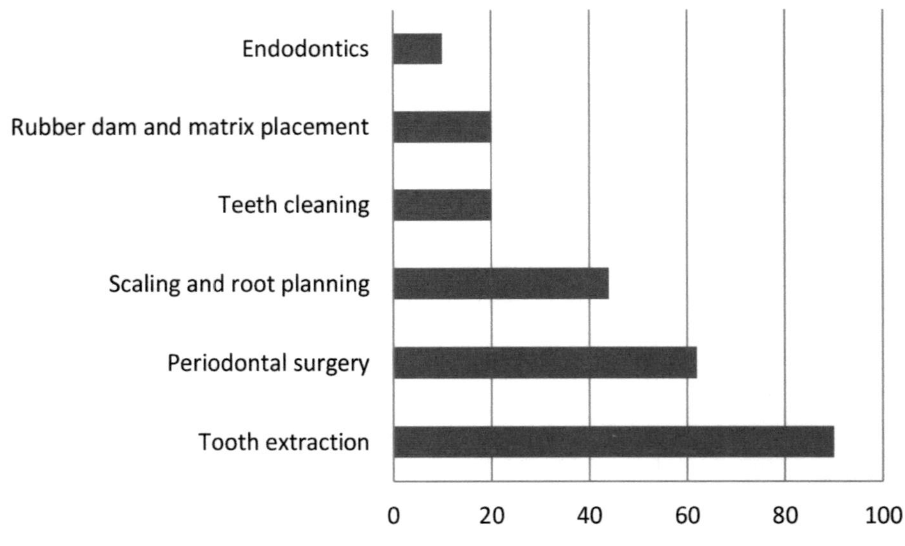

Figure 1. Prevalence of oral bacteraemia after dental procedures (inferred from [11]).

From early studies, it was generally accepted that the incidence and magnitude of bacteraemia of oral origin during dental procedures was directly proportional to the degree of inflammation and infection in the mouth. However, more recent series have found no relationship between the number of caries or the presence of periapical lesions and increased risk of post-intervention bacteraemia. Similarly, it is also accepted that the grade of gingival and periodontal health does not affect the presence or intensity of bacteraemia during interventions, and an increase in the prevalence of bacteraemia has only been demonstrated after tooth extractions in the setting of an acute infectious condition.

Studies that have investigated the bacteriological spectrum of bacteraemia of oral origin show a wide variability in their results due to the different sampling and detection techniques employed. However, *Streptococcus* spp.—the bacterial species most frequently implicated in IE of oral origin—is detected in at least 30% of cases [22]. This inoculum of streptococci that reaches the bloodstream has intrinsic pathogenic potential to colonise susceptible endocardial tissue in highest-risk patients. Structurally, streptococci have surface proteins (adhesins) that have been shown experimentally to have high affinity for the extracellular matrix, making the microorganisms capable of easily colonising vegetations and medical devices that become coated with matrix proteins after implantation. After colonisation, the bacterial biofilm acts as a propitious environment to perpetuate infection. The resulting fibrin and platelet deposition over the biofilm contributes to organise an actual bacteria-release clot which is able to create the recurrent bacteraemias that characterise IE.

A number of experimental studies have been able to reproduce these pathological events in animal models, but it remains to be seen whether oral bacteraemia secondary to dental interventions could promote identical results in humans [23].

A prospective study recently performed on patients diagnosed with IE appears to indicate that the mouth is a potential portal of entry (POE) for IE. A sample of 318 patients diagnosed with IE was examined prospectively by different specialists selected according to the natural habitat or site of colonisation of the causal diagnosed microorganism. A potential oral POE was detected by a stomatologist in 68 cases (21%), of which only 12% were considered possibly related to previous professional manipulation. Interestingly, the highest percentage of patients (88%) with oral and dental POEs was therefore made up of patients with no history of dental interventions. It was assumed that these patients presented a deficient state of oral health in the form of dental, endodontal or periodontal infection (**Table 7**).

These results agree strongly with those of Lockhart et al. [11] who presented a comparative study on the presence of bacteraemia in patients undergoing tooth extractions and toothbrushing. They found that the risk of oral bacteraemia was significantly associated with poor oral hygiene during toothbrushing. However, they did not find any association in the extraction group, even when performed without antibiotic cover. This is consistent with statements that patients at risk of IE have greater exposure to the action of oral bacteria during activities of daily living, such as toothbrushing or chewing, particularly if the individual has poor oral hygiene.

	N	%
Related to dental procedures (previous 3 months)	**8**	**12**
Tooth extraction	4	6
Scaling	1	1.5
Endodontics	1	1.5
No details	2	3
Not related to dental procedures	**60**	**88**
Dental focus of infection (decay, fracture, trauma)	9	13.3
Dental focus of infection (no further details)	22	32.1
Periodontal disease	7	10.3
Endodontal and periodontal disease	12	17.5
Radiological dental infectious focus with no clinical lesion	9	13.3
Vigorous tooth brushing with frequent bleeding	1	1.5

Table 7. Infective endocarditis patients with identified oral and dental portals of entry ($n = 68$) [24].

These observations highlight the importance of maintaining oral hygiene in patients at highest risk of IE, and provide an important argument that dental care could have greater repercussions than antibiotic prophylaxis on the incidence of IE of oral origin.

6. Evidence of the efficacy of antibiotic prophylaxis

Since the 1955 AHA statement, Ref. [2] antibiotic prophylaxis has been continuously recommended to clinicians for IE prevention among patients undergoing interventional medical procedures. Since that early paper, antibiotic prophylaxis for IE has been considered "good medical and dental practice" and it has been said that the "exact dosage and duration of therapy are somewhat empirical". Now, more than 50 years later, AHA experts continue to consider that the basis for the recommendations for IE prophylaxis are still not well established and that the quality of evidence is based on expert opinion, a few case-controlled studies, clinical experience and descriptive studies [11]. All these circumstances lead antibiotic prophylaxis against IE to be included in class C evidence (**Table 8**).

Level A	Data derived from multiple randomised clinical trials or meta-analyses
Level B	Data derived from a single randomised trial or non-randomised studies
Level C	Only expert consensus, case studies or standard of care

Table 8. Classification of the levels of evidence.

Despite this, intense research into this subject has been undertaken from three main perspectives:

- The prevention of bacterial endocarditis in experimental animal models.
- The efficacy of antibiotics for the prevention of bacteraemia secondary to dental procedures.
- Epidemiological studies.

6.1. The prevention of bacterial endocarditis in experimental animal models

The induction of IE in experimental animals was first achieved in 1970. The technique consisted of introducing a polyethylene catheter into the right side of the heart of the animal to induce a nonbacterial thrombotic endocarditis. Bacteria were then injected via the catheter to induce experimental bacterial endocarditis that served as a suitable model for the study of bacteriological, pathological and immunological aspects of IE [25].

Although experimental studies make it possible to investigate the efficacy of prophylactic antibiotic regimens against IE, there are difficulties associated with animal models both in their methodology and in the extrapolation of results. The plastic catheter acts as a foreign body delaying the successful treatment of established infection in animals, and the pharmacokinetics of antimicrobials in animals differ considerably from those in man [26].

The percentage of positive post-extraction blood cultures in experimental animals receiving antibiotic prophylaxis fell slightly with respect to the controls. However, it was observed that the administration of amoxicillin effectively prevented the onset of IE, allowing the researchers to suggest that the antibiotics had some protective mechanism over and above their bactericidal activity.

Animal research continues to be very useful for the preliminary evaluation of the efficacy and safety of drugs, and studies are being performed on the usefulness of other, alternative drugs to antibiotics for the prevention of IE in at-risk patients [27].

6.2. Efficacy of antibiotics in the prevention of bacteraemia secondary to dental procedures

The majority of studies show that amoxicillin is effective in the control of bacteraemia of oral origin, reducing the rate of positive blood cultures after dental interventions in a range that varies between 70 and 100%. There are a number of reports on the efficacy of alternative antibiotics to amoxicillin for the prevention of bacteraemia of oral origin. Results are heterogeneous as they are conditioned by numerous factors such as geographical situation, previous patient oral health status, blood culture sampling technique, microbiological analysis, resistance maps, etc.; however, in general, alternative antibiotics show a lower efficacy in the control of bacteraemia.

Interestingly, clindamycin constitutes the alternative antibiotic of choice to amoxicillin in the three main guidelines (AHA, ESC and AIEPEG). Although some studies have concluded that clindamycin was useful to reduce oral bacteraemia, more recently published studies have found that clindamycin prophylaxis does not produce a significant reduction in the incidence of oral bacteraemia during dental procedures [15, 28, 29]. Some authors have proposed moxifloxacin as an alternative to amoxicillin, given its efficacy in experimental endocarditis [30] and in the prevention of bacteraemia following dental procedures in humans [15]. However, endocarditis expert committees appear to be ignoring this antibiotic at the present time.

S. aureus is now the most common pathogen in IE. This circumstance could justify the use of amoxicillin in association with a β-lactamase inhibitor, such as clavulanate, to broaden the bactericidal spectrum of antibiotic prophylaxis against IE. A recent study suggests that intravenous amoxicillin/clavulanate could be effective in the prevention of oral bacteraemia, virtually eliminating post-procedure inocula [29]. This observation opens the door to further research into the efficacy of oral amoxicillin/clavulanate in the prevention of bacteraemia. In any case, given its unusual demonstrated effectiveness in the elimination of oral bacteraemia, the intravenous prophylactic regimen of amoxicillin/clavulanate could be a high-efficacy alternative for patients with cardiac risk factors and severe systemic alterations, such as immune compromise, who require curative interventional dental treatment.

6.3. Epidemiological studies

Up to 2008, epidemiological studies did not support the hypothesis for the use of prophylactic antibiotics for medical procedures as a preventive method against IE. Case-control studies indicated that most IE events occurred independently of medical interventions and of the administration of antibiotic prophylaxis. A further argument was that despite the universal application of antibiotic prophylaxis, the incidence of IE and its associated mortality had not varied over decades [5].

In 2008, cessation of the NICE recommendation for antibiotic prophylaxis introduced a new epidemiological context into the study of IE, and analysis will serve to establish reliable conclusions in its area of influence. Implementation of the NICE guideline in England provides an opportunity for retrospective studies to investigate the comparative effect of antibiotic prophylaxis versus no prophylaxis on the incidence of IE.

Initially, the data suggest a significant increase in the incidence of IE after implantation of the NICE guideline, rising above the projected historical trend. This observation could lead to the hypothesis that the increased incidence of IE could be related to medical procedures in susceptible individuals performed without appropriate antibiotic cover. With regard to the dental procedures, we should observe an increase in the incidence of IE caused by oral viridans group streptococci but, at the present time, no data are available on pathogen-specific causal microorganisms [30].

7. Detractors of antibiotic prophylaxis

In view of the lack of scientific evidence on the prophylactic efficacy of the antibiotics for the prevention of IE, the British health authorities have focused their attention on the principle problems of the indiscriminate administration of antibiotics [6]:

http://dx.doi.org/10.5772/65255

- Quantifiable risk to the individual patient.
- Creation of unnecessary antimicrobial resistance.
- Economic burden.

However, a recent study on the incidence and nature of adverse reactions to antibiotics prescribed for endocarditis prophylaxis in England from 2004 estimates that reported adverse drug reaction rates from amoxicillin prescribed as antibiotic prophylaxis are low, without a single fatal reaction for nearly 3 million prescriptions [31].

The emergence of antibiotic resistance is a serious public health problem, but prophylactic antibiotic regimens for IE would only have a very limited effect as evidence shows that bacteria acquire resistance to antibiotics only after the administration of several consecutive doses.

With regard to the cost to the national health systems of the systematic administration of prophylaxis, cost-efficacy analyses of antibiotic prophylaxis for at-risk patients undergoing dental treatment provided contradictory results. In some countries, such as the USA, it has been estimated that prophylaxis constitutes a considerable expense, [32] but their results cannot be extrapolated to other countries in which the administration of prophylactic antibiotics to high-risk patients only represents a very small percentage of all the antibiotics that dentists prescribe.

Research into the control of bacteraemia shows that the administration of amoxicillin significantly reduces bacteraemia of oral origin, though it does not completely eliminate the possibility that this could occur. Alternative antibiotics such as clindamycin have shown poor results in the reduction of bacteraemia after dental interventions, leading us to deduce that the efficacy of prophylactic antibiotics in the prevention of IE in high-risk patients undergoing dental manipulations is limited.

8. Future research

Studies published to date on antibiotic prophylaxis against IE have a series of limitations that hinder their extrapolation, and attention must be focused on this aspect in future research:

- Regarding participants, it has been suggested that the prevalence of post-extraction bacteraemia may be related to age [33]. Age is also a determining factor in the pharmacokinetics of the antibiotic, and the efficacy of specific prophylaxis regimens may differ between children and adults. The oral health status may also influence the prevalence of post-dental manipulation bacteraemia, although this is still a controversial issue [34].
- The mode of anaesthesia, particularly general anaesthesia, can determine the appearance of post-extraction bacteraemia and prolong its duration. Comparative studies should therefore be performed using local and general anaesthesia [35].

- The prevalence of bacteraemia secondary to dental treatment and probably the predominant bacterial species are determined by the nature of the procedure. We therefore do not know whether antibiotic prophylaxis will be equally effective for different dental procedures [22].
- It is not known whether the dose and route of administration for the majority of current antibiotic prophylaxis regimens has a bearing on antibacterial activity.
- The fact that positive post-dental-manipulation blood cultures are not detected after the administration of antibiotic prophylaxis does not guarantee that bacteraemia does not occur due to bacteria that cannot be cultured in the usual culture media and/or whose inoculum is below the threshold of the method of detection employed.

Author details

Miguel Castro, Javier Álvarez, Javier F. Feijoo, Marcio Diniz, Lucía García-Caballero, Pedro Diz* and Jacobo Limeres

*Address all correspondence to: pedro.diz@usc.es

Special Needs Unit and OMEQUI Research Group, School of Medicine and Dentistry, Santiago de Compostela University, Santiago de Compostela, Spain

References

[1] Elliot SD. Bacteraemia and oral sepsis. Proc R Soc Med 1939; 32: 747–754.

[2] American Heart Association. Prevention of rheumatic fever and bacterial endocarditis through control of streptococcal infections. Circulation 1955; 11: 317–320.

[3] Pelletier LL Jr, Durack DT, Petersdorf RG. Chemotherapy of experimental streptococcal endocarditis. IV. Further observations on prophylaxis. J Clin Invest 1975; 56: 319–330.

[4] British Society for Antimicrobial Chemotherapy. The antibiotic prophylaxis of infective endocarditis. Lancet 1982; 2: 1323–1326.

[5] Prendergast BD. The changing face of infective endocarditis. Heart 2006; 92: 879–885.

[6] National Institute for Health and Clinical Excellence. Prophylaxis against infective endocarditis. Antimicrobial prophylaxis against infective endocarditis in adults and children undergoing interventional procedures 2008. http://nice.org.uk/CG064

[7] Thornhill MH, Dayer MJ, Forde JM, et al. Impact of the NICE guideline recommending cessation of antibiotic prophylaxis for prevention of infective endocarditis: before and after study. BMJ 2011; 342: d2392.

[8] Lopez R, Flavell S, Thomas C. A not very NICE case of endocarditis. BMJ Case Rep 2013: bcr2012007918.

[9] Dayer MJ, Jones S, Prendergast B, Baddour LM, Lockhart PB, Thornhill MH. Incidence of infective endocarditis in England, 2000–2013: a secular trend, interrupted time-series analysis. Lancet 2015; 385: 1219–1228.

[10] Thornhill MH, Dayer M, Lockhart PB, et al. Guidelines on prophylaxis to prevent infective endocarditis. Br Dent J 2016; 220: 51–56.

[11] Wilson W, Taubert KA, Gewitz M, et al. Prevention of infective endocarditis. Guidelines from the American Heart Association. J Am Dent Assoc 2007; 138: 739–745, 747–760.

[12] Moulds RF, Jeyasingham MS. Infective Endocarditis Prophylaxis Expert Group, Therapeutic Guidelines Limited. Antibiotic prophylaxis against infective endocarditis: time to rethink. Med J Aust 2008; 189: 301–302.

[13] Habib G, Lancellotti P, Antunes MJ, et al. 2015 ESC Guidelines for the management of infective endocarditis: the task force for the management of infective endocarditis of the European Society of Cardiology (ESC). Endorsed by: European Association for Cardio-Thoracic Surgery (EACTS), the European Association of Nuclear Medicine (EANM). Eur Heart J 2015; 36: 3075–3128.

[14] Becker DE. Drug allergies and implications for dental practice. Anesth Prog 2013 Winter; 60: 188–197.

[15] Diz Dios P, Tomás Carmona I, Limeres Posse J, Medina Henríquez J, Fernández Feijoo J, Álvarez Fernández M. Comparative efficacies of amoxicillin, clindamycin, and moxifloxacin in prevention of bacteremia following dental extractions. Antimicrob Agents Chemother 2006; 50: 2996–3002.

[16] Addy LD, Martin MV. Azithromycin and dentistry—a useful agent?. Br Dent J 2004; 197: 141–143.

[17] Vogkou CT, Vlachogiannis NI, Palaiodimos L, Kousoulis AA. The causative agents in infective endocarditis: a systematic review comprising 33,214 cases. Eur J Clin Microbiol Infect Dis 2016; 35: 1227–1245.

[18] Dajani AS, Taubert KA, Wilson W, et al. Prevention of bacterial endocarditis: recommendations by the American Heart Association. Clin Infect Dis 1997; 25: 1448–1458.

[19] Davies SB, Hofer A, Reeve C. Mortality attributable to rheumatic heart disease in the Kimberley: a data linkage approach. Intern Med J 2014; 44: 1074–1080.

[20] Lockhart PB, Loven B, Brennan MT, Fox PC. The evidence base for the efficacy of antibiotic prophylaxis in dental practice. J Am Dent Assoc 2007; 138: 458–474.

[21] Okell CC, Elliott SD. Bacteraemia and oral sepsis with special reference to subacute endocarditis. Lancet 1935; 226: 869–887.

[22] Diz Dios P, Tomás Carmona I, Limeres Posse J. ***Bateriemias producidas por intervenciones odontológicas (chap. 13). In: Patología Periodontal y Cardiovascular. Coordinators: De Teresa E, Noguerol Rodríguez B. Editorial: Panamericana S.A., Madrid, 2011: 159–167.

[23] Veloso TR, Amiguet M, Rousson V, et al. Induction of experimental endocarditis by continuous low-grade bacteremia mimicking spontaneous bacteremia in humans. Infect Immun 2011; 79: 2006–2011.

[24] Delahaye F, M'Hammedi A, Guerpillon B, et al. Systematic search for present and potential portals of entry for infective endocarditis. J Am Coll Cardiol 2016; 67: 151–158.

[25] Garrison PK, Freedman LR. Experimental endocarditis I. *Staphylococcal endocarditis* in rabbits resulting from placement of a polyethylene catheter in the right side of the heart. Yale J Biol Med 1970; 42: 394–410.

[26] Petersdorf RG. Antimicrobial prophylaxis of bacterial endocarditis. Prudent caution or bacterial overkill? Am J Med 1978; 65: 220–223.

[27] Veloso TR, Mancini S, Giddey M, et al. Vaccination against *Staphylococcus aureus* experimental endocarditis using recombinant *Lactococcus lactis* expressing ClfA or FnbpA. Vaccine 2015; 33: 3512–3517.

[28] Maharaj B, Coovadia Y, Vayej AC. A comparative study of amoxicillin, clindamycin and chlorhexidine in the prevention of post-extraction bacteraemia. Cardiovasc J Afr 2012; 23: 491–494.

[29] Limeres Posse J, Álvarez Fernández M, Fernández Feijoo J, et al. Intravenous amoxicillin/clavulanate for the prevention of bacteraemia following dental procedures: a randomized clinical trial. J Antimicrob Chemother 2016; 71: 2022–2030.

[30] Sakka V, Galani L, Pefanis A, et al. Successful moxifloxacin prophylaxis against experimental streptococcal aortic valve endocarditis. J Antimicrob Chemother 2005; 56: 1160–1162.

[31] Thornhill MH, Dayer MJ, Prendergast B, Baddour LM, Jones S, Lockhart PB. Incidence and nature of adverse reactions to antibiotics used as endocarditis prophylaxis. J Antimicrob Chemother 2015; 70: 2382–2388.

[32] Lockhart PB, Blizzard J, Maslow AL, Brennan MT, Sasser H, Carew J. Drug cost implications for antibiotic prophylaxis for dental procedures. Oral Surg Oral Med Oral Pathol Oral Radiol 2013; 115: 345–353.

[33] Lockhart PB, Brennan MT, Kent ML, Norton HJ, Weinrib DA. Impact of amoxicillin prophylaxis on the incidence, nature, and duration of bacteremia in children after intubation and dental procedures. Circulation 2004; 109: 2878–2884.

http://dx.doi.org/10.5772/65255

[34] Lockhart PB, Brennan MT, Thornhill M, et al. Poor oral hygiene as a risk factor for infective endocarditis-related bacteremia. J Am Dent Assoc 2009; 140: 1238–1244.

[35] Barbosa M, Carmona IT, Amaral B, et al. General anesthesia increases the risk of bacteremia following dental extractions. Oral Surg Oral Med Oral Pathol Oral Radiol Endod 2010; 110: 706–712.

Chapter 3

Epidemiology of Infective Endocarditis

Fabian Andres Giraldo Vallejo

Additional information is available at the end of the chapter

http://dx.doi.org/10.5772/65030

Abstract

Infective endocarditis is a rare disease, with an incidence of two to six episodes per 100,000 habitants/year. Incidence is higher in elderly people; besides, this group is often affected by many comorbidities. There is a clear and observable change in the spectrum of heart diseases predisposing to infective endocarditis in the last decades. Up to one-third of the patients acquire the disease on a health-care-associated environment. Despite advances in health-care logistics, infective endocarditis remains a big concern especially in low-income countries, where the main cause of infection is rheumatic fever. In-hospital mortality persists relatively high despite development in medical and surgical treatment. Patients with infective endocarditis need rapid response and prompt diagnosis from a multidisciplinary group including cardiologists, surgeons, infectologists, and radiologists.

Keywords: endocarditis, epidemiology, microbiology, outcome, incidence, mortality

1. Introduction

The term *infective endocarditis* (IE) denotes infection of the endocardial surface of the heart. Infection involves heart valves most commonly but may occur within a septal defect, chordae tendinae, or in the mural endocardium. Infections of arteriovenous shunts, arterioarterial shunts (patent ductus arteriosus), or coarctation of the aorta are clinically and pathologically similar to IE. The characteristic lesion of the IE, the vegetation, is a variably sized mass with inflammatory cells, platelets, fibrin, and abundant immerse microorganisms. The term *infective endocarditis,* first used by Thayer and later popularized by Lerner and Weinstein,is preferable to the former term bacterial endocarditis, because chlamydiae, rickettsiae, mycoplasmas, fungi, and perhaps even viruses may be responsible for the syndrome [1].

Diagnostic criteria for IE were published in 1982 by von Reyn and colleagues (The Beth Israel criteria), but these criteria did not use echocardiographic findings in the case definitions [2]. Including the central role of echocardiography in the evaluation of suspected IE, new case definitions and diagnostic criteria (The Duke criteria) were proposed in 1994 [3], modified in 2000, and widely used since then (**Table 1**) [4]. Echocardiography utility in the diagnosis of IE is clearly recognized [5], transesophageal imaging has superior sensitivity and specificity, is cost-effective, and is recommended when transthoracic approach is negative and a high clinical suspicion is present. The utility of both modalities is diminished when used indiscriminately [6, 7]. Advances in imaging technology have had minimal impact at the day-to-day clinical level; the role of three-dimensional (3D) echocardiography and other modes of clinical imaging (magnetic resonance imaging, computed tomography, and technetium scintigraphy) are yet to be formally evaluated [8].

Definition of infective endocarditis (IE) according to modified Duke criteria

Definite infective endocarditis

Pathologic criteria

- **Microorganisms demonstrated by culture or histologic examination of a vegetation, a vegetation that has embolized, or an intracardiac abscess specimen;** ***or***
- **Pathologic lesions; vegetation or intracardiac abscess confirmed by histologic examination showing active endocarditis**

Clinical criteria

- **Two major criteria;** ***or***
- **One major criterion and three minor criteria;** ***or***
- **Five minor criteria**

Possible infective endocarditis

- **One major criterion and one minor criterion;** ***or***
- **Three minor criteria**

Rejected

- **Firm alternate diagnosis explaining evidence of IE;** ***or***
- **Resolution of IE syndrome with antibiotic therapy for ≤4 days;** ***or***
- **No pathologic evidence of IE at surgery or autopsy, with antibiotic therapy for ≤4 days;** ***or***
- **Does not meet criteria for possible IE, as above**

Major criteria

Blood culture positive for IE

- **Typical microorganisms consistent with IE from two separate blood cultures: viridans** ***Streptococci, Streptococcus bovis*****, HACEK group,** ***Staphylococcus aureus; or***

- **Community-acquired *Enterococci*, in the absence of a primary focus; *or***
- **Microorganisms consistent with IE from persistently positive blood cultures, defined as follows:**
- **At least two positive cultures of blood samples drawn >12 h apart; *or***
- **All of three or a majority of ≥ four separate cultures of blood (with first and last sample drawn at least 1 h apart)**
- **Single positive blood culture for *Coxiella burnetii* or antiphase I IgG antibody titer >1:800**

Evidence of endocardial involvement

- **Echocardiogram positive for IE (TEE recommended in patients with prosthetic valves, rated at least "possible IE" by clinical criteria, or complicated IE (paravalvular abscess); TTE as first test in other patients), defined as follows:**
    - **Oscillating intracardiac mass on valve or supporting structures, in the path of regurgitant jets, or on implanted material in the absence of an alternative anatomic explanation; *or***
    - **Abscess; *or***
    - **New partial dehiscence of prosthetic valve New valvular regurgitation (worsening or changing of preexisting murmur not sufficient)**

Minor criteria

- **Predisposition, predisposing heart condition or injection drug use**
- **Fever, temperature >38·C (100.4·F)**
- **Vascular phenomena, major arterial emboli, septic pulmonary infarcts, mycotic aneurysm, intracranial hemorrhage, conjunctival hemorrhages, and Janeway lesions**
- **Immunologic phenomena: glomerulonephritis, Osler's nodes, Roth's spots, and rheumatoid factor**
- **Microbiologic evidence: positive blood culture but does not meet a major criterion as noted above* or serologic evidence of active infection with organism consistent with IE**
- **Echocardiographic minor criteria eliminated**

TEE, transesophageal echocardiography; TTE, transthoracic echocardiography. Modified from [4].

Table 1. HACEK, *Hemophilus* spp., *Aggregatibacter* spp., *Cardiobacterium hominis, Eikenella corrodens,* and *Kingella* spp.

The challenges associated with IE are of increasing importance. The patients affected are older and sicker than those in the past, often with many comorbidities [9]. *Staphylococcus aureus* has surpassed penicillin-sensitive *Streptococci* as the most common cause in many high-income countries [10]. The population at risk is growing and health-care-associated *Staphylococcal bacteremia*, a conditioning of IE, is a major problem around the world [11].

In the last 30 years, the overall incidence of IE has remained between two and six per 100,000 individuals per year in the general population [12–14], whereas associated mortality has remained between 10 and 30% depending on the type of pathogen [15], the site of infection (native or prosthetic valve), and the underlying condition [16]. This quiescent trends in mortality and incidence are due to a continuing evolution of epidemiological features and risk factors rather to a lack of medical progress. The variability of disease presentation and course represents a challenge for the physician [8]. Even though clinical practices are clearly explained by international guides, they are derived mainly from observational cohort studies rather than randomized trials [17, 18]. Chronic rheumatic heart disease was considered a primary risk factor for IE until the widespread introduction of antibiotics; nevertheless, this finding prevails for low-income countries [14]. Current behavior in industrialized countries portraits different risk groups including prosthetic valve recipients, intravenous (IV) drug users, individuals with intravenous catheters, patients undergoing hemodialysis, and elderly people with degenerative valve lesions. Oral *Streptococci* are the main cause of IE in the general population [14, 19, 20], whereas *S. aureus* and coagulase-negative *Staphylococci* (e.g., *S. epidermidis*) are more frequently found in intravenous drug users, individuals with prosthetic-valve IE and in those with health-care-related IE [12, 21–23] and group *D Streptococci* (e.g. *S. gallolyticus*) are increasingly prevalent in elderly patients [12, 14, 19, 24, 25]. Patients with IE require opportune diagnosis and prompt response from a multidisciplinary group including cardiologists, cardiac surgeons, infectious disease specialists, and radiologists. The logistics of high-level patient care remains difficult even in developed countries and is frequently unobtainable in low-income countries.

2. Epidemiology

The incidence of IE is difficult to determine, because the diagnosis criteria and reporting methods vary with different series [2, 26]. The annual incidence of IE reported in Olmsted County, MN, was five to seven cases per 100,000 person-years, from 1970 to 2000, with practically no change in this period interval [27]. Parallel results of 1.7 per 100,000 person-years were reported from a survey in Louisiana [28], similar to reports from France (2.4/100,000 person-year) [19, 29] and United Kingdom [30]. But these results are less than incidence reports from the Delaware river Valley region (11.6/100,000 population) [31]. Several series have reported considerable increments in hospitalizations for IE, with most of the increase ascribable to *S. aureus* [32]. The proportion of acute cases of IE has increased from approximately 20% in the pre-antibiotic era, to more than 75% in the majority of high-income countries today [9].

When investigating at IE history, it can be seen that it affected children and young adults as a result of chronic rheumatic heart disease [33]; nevertheless, this remains the first key factor for IE in developing countries representing up to two-thirds of cases [34, 35] and infection is caused predominantly by community-acquired, penicillin-sensitive *Streptococci* entering via the oral cavity. The mean age of patients with IE has increased gradually in the antibiotic era. In 1926, the median age was younger than 30 years [36]; by 1943, it was 39 years [25], 50 years in the 1980s, and 55–60 years in the 1990s and 2000s [2, 12, 13, 19]. In a recent report including 58 centers in 25 countries, covering more than 2700 patients with definite IE by modified Duke criteria, the median age was 57.9 year [9]. In the period from 1993 to 2003, including 3784 patients with IE, the incidence of infection was <5 per 100,000 patients per year in individuals aged 50 years or less and >15 per 100,000 patients per year in those older

http://dx.doi.org/10.5772/65030

than 65 years [12]. In a recent review comprising 3477 patients, the mean age of individuals with IE in 1980s was 45.3 years versus 57.2 years in 2000s [37]. These increasing rates of IE in the elderly could be the accumulation of factors such as improved living standards, which indirectly increase the population with degenerative valve disease hence leading to increasingly prosthetic valve surgeries in older patients. More men are affected than women; 58.6% in 1970s versus 66.3% in 2000s [37]. In a French study, the incidence of IE increased in patients older than 50 years and peaked at 194 infected per million habitants in men aged 75–79 years (**Figure 1**) [10].

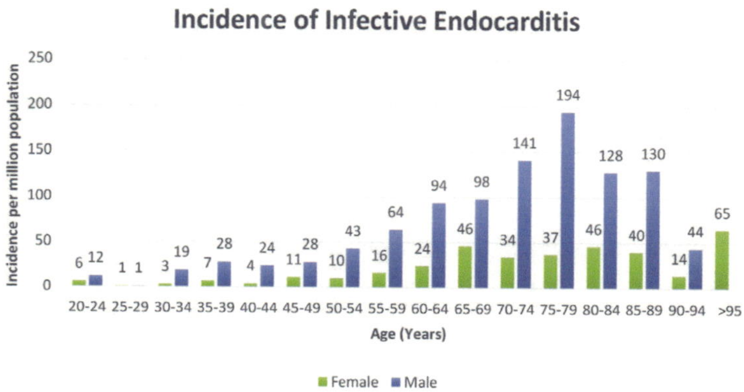

Figure 1. Incidence of infective endocarditis according to age and sex in a French population study of 497 patients. Zenith at 194 cases per million in men aged 75–79 years. Adapted from Selton-Suty et al. [10].

The causative agent has not changed much over time: *Staphylococci* spp., *Streptococci* spp., and *Enterococci* spp. still comprising more than 80% of all cases. Among these, *S. aureus* exceeds *Streptococci* spp. by 12% (**Figure 2**) [9].

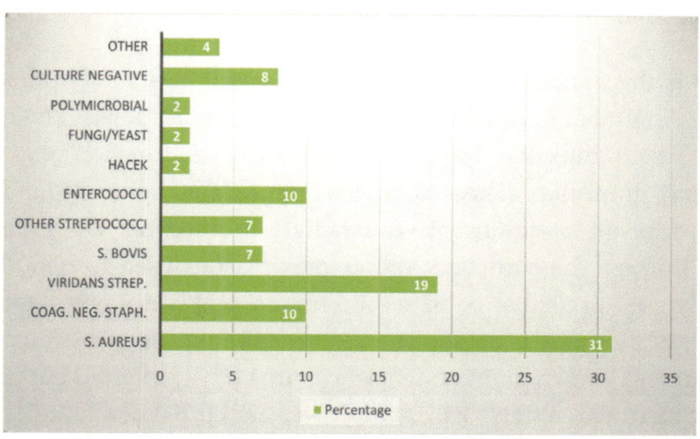

Figure 2. Microbiologic etiology of endocarditis in 1558 patients. Fifty-eight hospitals in 25 countries between June 2000 and September 2005. Data from Murdoch DR, Corey CR, Hoen B., et al. [9]

2.1. Health-care-associated endocarditis

Owing to introduction of new therapeutic modalities (e.g., pacemakers, intravenous catheters, hyperalimentation lines, and dialysis shunts), health-care-associated IE, a relatively new form of the disease, has emerged [2, 9, 22, 23, 38–40]. Health-care-associated endocarditis includes nosocomial IE as well as community IE after a recent hospitalization or as a consequence of long-term indwelling devices. In a recent prospective, multinational cohort study from 61 hospitals in 28 countries comprising 1622 patients with native valve endocarditis (NVE), and no intravenous drug abuse, 34% of patients had health-care-associated endocarditis with nearly half being community acquired [40]. Infection may compromise normal valves, including the tricuspid valve, as well as implanted intracardiac devices and valves [9, 21, 40–43]. The heart valve involved by infection varies considerably according to the different series. For mitral valve alone, the distribution ranges from 28 to 45%, aortic valve alone 5–36%, and aortic and mitral combined 0–35%. The tricuspid valve rarely is involved ranging from 0 to 6% and even less the pulmonary valve (<1%) [9, 44]. Health-care-associated IE accounts for 24 to 34% of cases not related to current cardiac surgery, and it involves an even larger proportion of cases in the United States [9, 23, 40]. Proportion of health-care-associated native valve endocarditis is 54% for nosocomial cases and 46% for community-based cases [40]. Mortality rates among these patients are high, ranging from 27 to 38%; aggravating factors include older patients and complex comorbidities [40, 41]. Among patients with health-care-associated IE, the largest subgroup belongs to individuals undergoing hemodialysis [22, 45]. Chronic hemodialysis has been identified as an independent risk factor for this type of IE [22, 40]. Patients undergoing hemodialysis have a higher risk of *S. aureus* infection causing IE [40, 45, 46]. The two most common pathogens related to health-care-associated IE are *Staphylococci* and *Enterococci*; the infection usually originates in the urinary tract or skin and intravenous lines or invasive procedures are often identified [40]. The risk of IE can be as high as 10% in cases of catheter-induced *S. aureus* bacteremia [39, 47, 48].

2.2. Immunocompromised patient IE

A special group is the immunocompromised patient who has a suboptimally functioning immune system. A number of conditions alter the immune response. The elderly has weak bactericidal response to infection. Impaired B-cell and T-cell function may develop in poor nutrition status or malnutrition. Hematologic and lymphoid malignancies and the medications used to treat them result in significant vulnerability to infection. The immune response is further reduced through the corticoids and cytotoxic drugs used to treat these conditions. Radiation therapy used to treat or palliate solid tumors and lymphoma suppresses antibody formation for weeks after treatment [49]. The degree of immunosuppression plays a major role in the outcome among human immunodeficiency virus (HIV)-infected patients with IE. Poor outcome is associated with a CD4+ cell count lower than 0.200 per 10(9)/L and left-sided or mixed IE [50, 51]. Common organisms associated with IE in HIV-infected patients are *S. aureus* and *Salmonella* [52]. Fungal microorganisms such as *Candida albicans, Aspergillus,* and *Cryptococcus neoformans* are more common in IV drug abusers with HIV. These patients possess a greater risk of developing IE on the right-sided heart valves [52]. Infection with HIV should not preclude cardiac surgery.

2.3. Prosthetic valve endocarditis.

Different series suggest that prosthetic valve endocarditis (PVE) accounts for 10–30% of cases of IE in the developed world [23, 41, 53, 54]. In patients undergoing valve surgery between 1965 and 1995, the cumulative incidence of PVE ranged from 1.4 to 3.1% at 12 months and 3 to 5.7% at 5 years [42]. Associated risks for the development of PVE include male sex, previous native valve compromise, and long cardiopulmonary bypass for prosthetic valve placement [55]. Microbial seeding may occur in the early postimplantation period, before endothelialization has established. The incidence is greatest in the first 6 months after valve surgery, then declines to a lower but stable rate (0.2–0.35% per year) [56–58]. The range of age of PVE patients varies from 50 to 74 years [19, 43, 53, 59–62]. The risk of PVE is higher when valve replacement is performed during active IE, especially with unknown pathogen or incomplete antibiotic treatment [58, 63–66]. Mechanical prostheses seem to have a slightly higher risk for PVE in the first 3 months after implantation and bioprosthetic valves have a higher risk after 1 year of replacement [56, 64, 65], maybe as a result of degeneration of bioprosthetic leaflets. Although the cumulative risk comparing mechanical with biological prosthesis is similar [42, 67, 68], the weighted mean incidence for infections of bioprostheses calculated from different series is 0.49% per patient-year for mitral valves and 0.91% per patient-year for aortic valves. For mechanical prostheses, the incidence is 0.18% per patient-year for mitral, 0.27% per patient-year for aortic, and 0.29% per patient-year for multiple implants [63]. PVE has been called *early* when infection occurred within 2 months of valve surgery and *late* when onset was >2 months. These terms were established to help distinguish PVE that instituted early as a complication of valve surgery from tardy infection that was likely to be community acquired [58, 69, 70]. However, in 2007, a study demonstrated a major shift according to the biological profile at 12 months after surgery, indicating that a more appropriate cutoff time to distinguish early from late PVE was 1 year [71]. Moreover, the European guidelines use this limit to classify the condition [17]. The causative pathogens involved in early PVE usually are methicillin-resistant *Staphylococci,* whereas in late PVE the common pathogens found are coagulase-negative *Staphylococci* and *Enterococci* (**Table 2**) [53]. In a large series including 2572 patients who underwent transcatheter aortic valve replacement (TAVR) in 14 centers between January 2008 and April 2013, the incidence of TAVR PVE was 1.13% (29 patients); the incidence of TAVR PVE by transfemoral approach was 1.1%, transapical 1.98%. The incidence of IE was 1.93% for balloon-expandable (23 of 1191) and 0.45% (6 of 1343) for self-expandable transcatheter heart valves. Early-onset IE (within 60 days) was diagnosed in 28% (eight patients), intermediate-onset IE (between 60 and 265 days) was diagnosed in 52% (15 patients), and late-onset IE (>1 year) was diagnosed in 20% (six patients) resulting in 80% of incidence of IE within the first 12 months of implantation (higher rates), contrasting with surgical valve IE. In the early-onset group, *S. aureus* and coagulase-negative *Staphylococci* were the most prevalent (50%); in the intermediate-onset group *Staphylococcal, Enterococcal,* and *non-viridans Streptococcal* species were the predominant pathogens (20% each), and in the late-onset group *Staphylococci* and *Enterococci* were identified (33% each), which does not resemble the late-onset surgical PVE [72].

PATHOGEN	EARLY PVE* (%) *N* = 53	LATE PVE* (%) *N* = 331
Staphylococcus aureus	36	18
Coagulase-negative Staphylococci	17	20
Enterococcus	8	13
Viridans streptococci	2	10
Streptococcus bovis	2	7
HACEK	0	2
Fungi	9	3
Other	6	14
Culture negative	17	12

Adapted from Wang et al. [53]. *Early refers to IE within 2 months and late after 2 months, according to Wang et al. HACEK: *Hemophilus, Aggregatibacter spp., Cardiobacterium hominis, Eikenella corrodens, Kingella kingae.* PVE: Prosthetic valve endocarditis.

Table 2. Causative organisms for early and late PVE.

2.4. Cardiovascular-implantable electronic devices infection

The most commonly used cardiovascular-implantable electronic device (CIED) are permanent pacemaker, cardiac resynchronization therapy, and implantable cardioverter-defibrillator. Most of these are implanted using transvenous leads. This practice had dramatically reduced the risk of infection associated with the procedure. Nevertheless, complication by infection remains a problem that can lead to significant morbidity, mortality, and elevated costs [73–75]. Reports of CIED infection vary according to different series and range from 0.13 to 19.9% [76–78]. In a 16-year survey of Nationwide Inpatient Sample (NIS) from 1993 to 2008, the rate of CIED implantation increased 4.7% annually. The incidence of CIED infection remained stable until 2004, but increased almost twice in a 4-year period (2004–2008) from 1.53 to 2.41%, respectively [75]. The rate of infection associated with implantable cardioverter-defibrillator surpasses greatly that of the pacemaker [79–81].

2.5. Ventricular-assist devices infection

Patients who receive ventricular-assist devices (VADs) usually have various comorbidities, including a state of immune compromise. The risk of infection varies depending on the duration of VAD support [82]. Higher rates of infection are observed in the destination therapy group compared with the group where VAD is used as a bridge to transplantation [82]. Hravnak reported that registry patients with implant duration longer than 60 days were twice as likely to develop infection than those patients supported for less than 30 days [83]. The reported rates of infection in patients with VAD range from 13 to 80% and depend on multiple factors, including comorbidities, type of device implanted, and duration of VAD support [84]. Infection of VAD can present as three different syndromes: driveline infection (most frequent) presenting with local inflammatory changes and drainage at exit site, pocket site infection is the second syndrome presenting with local inflammatory changes, and the third (least frequent) is endocarditis comprising valves and/or internal lining of the device [84].

2.6. Infection of closure devices (atrial septal defect, patent ductus arteriosus, and ventricular septal defect)

Minimally invasive procedures are increasingly accepted as an option for cardiovascular congenital diseases [85–87]. Fortunately, complications derived from implantation of such devices are very rare, including infection (<1%) [85, 88–90].

2.7. Infective endocarditis in children

As in adults, trends in children IE are related to the evolution of care in the sick child, particularly children born with congenital heart disease. The incidence of children IE provides limited data, mostly based on inpatient admission which could not represent accurately the general population. In a report between 1933 and 1972, the incidence was 0.22–0.55 cases per 1000 pediatric hospital admissions [91]. A retrospective review between 1972 and 1982 found an incidence of 1/1280 pediatric admissions [92]. Later, in a multicenter study, the incidence of IE slightly decreased, ranging from 0.005 to 0.12 cases per 1000 pediatric admissions [93]. In other report including 47,518 patients, from 1998 to 2010, congenital heart disease was found as the major underlying condition associated to IE in children in high-income countries, with a cumulative incidence of 6.1 per 1000 children [94]. The distribution of IE between boys and girls is balanced in contrast with series in adults in whom men have a higher tendency to suffer the condition [94, 95]. Rheumatic fever is rare in developed countries, nevertheless is commonly found in low-income countries. In the presurgical era, the proportion of IE in children with rheumatic heart disease ranged from 30 to 50% [96]. A single center report covering seven decades found that IE occurred in 31% of rheumatic heart disease patients in presurgical era, compared to era 3 (1992–2004) with only 1.1% of patients having the condition [97]. Approximately 50% of cases of pediatric IE complicating congenital heart disease have had previous cardiac surgery, especially palliative shunts of complex cardiac repair [98]. Risk of postoperative IE in children depends greatly on the type of surgery; for example, a study from Oregon found a relatively low incidence of IE after tetralogy of Fallot repair (1.3%), ventricular septal repair (2.7%), atrial septal repair (2.8%), and aortic coarctation repair (3.5%). Nevertheless, a high incidence of IE was found in aortic stenosis (valve replacement) with a cumulative incidence at 25 years of 13.3% [99]. The rate of IE in structurally normal hearts is lower than those with a predisposing condition (22 vs. 78%), respectively [100]. A major risk factor to develop IE in an anatomically normal heart is an indwelling vascular catheter [101].

2.8. Infective endocarditis in adults

An important condition related to IE in the elderly is the congenital bicuspid aortic valve. In a prospective multicenter study, it was present in 16% of cases of native valve endocarditis [102]. Degenerative cardiac lesions assume an important role in the development of IE without underlying valve disease. In one study, degenerative lesions were present in 50% of patients with native valve IE older than 60 years [103]. Calcified mitral annulus is a common finding in elderly women but rarely complicate with IE (3.8%) [104]. Even not a classical condition related to IE, idiopathic hypertrophic subaortic stenosis may represent up to 5% of incidence of the infection [105]. And there is a higher mortality rate correlation if a murmur is present (up to 36% of patients with hypertrophic aortic stenosis and IE) [105]. Another condition associated with IE is the mitral prolapse syndrome. In different series, the range of IE in those patients with mitral valve prolapse can go from 11 to 23% [106, 107]. In another study, 8.6% of patients with mitral valve prolapse who were monitored prospectively for 9–22 years developed IE [108]. This syndrome must be suspected in patients with mid-systolic click with or without a late systolic murmur. This condition is not uncommon and has been found in 0.5–20% of otherwise healthy people, especially young women. It has become apparent that a significant proportion of patients with mitral valve prolapse have an anthropometrically distinct habitus, suggesting that this condition is only an element of a generalized developmental syndrome [109]. It may be useful to have in mind these characteristics to help identify patients with a high risk of developing IE. Having valvular redundancy and thickened leaflets may increase the risk of IE [103]. The combination of mitral valve prolapse and men older than 45 years also may increase the risk of IE [110]. In a detailed case-control study, 25% of patients with IE had mitral valve prolapse; the odds ratio (8.2 of 95% confidence interval, 2.4–28.4) indicated a substantially higher risk for IE in patients with mitral valve prolapse than for those without it [111]. Another study found that mitral valve prolapse IE presented with more subtle symptoms, less mortality, and responded better to antimicrobial therapy than other types of left-sided IE, even though recognition of the infection was delayed [112].

2.9. Infective endocarditis in drug abusers

All estimations of IE incidence in drug abusers are hindered because there are no enough data reporting the exact number of victims of illicit drug-abuse epidemic. Reports from the United States present an incidence of IE in intravenous drug abusers that range from 2 to 5% per year [113] or 1.5–2 cases per 1000 years of IV drug abuse with men more commonly affected [114]. Although congenital cardiac disease and right-sided heart instrumentation are associated with IE, IV drug abusers retain the majority of cases. Intravenous drug users and those with HIV primarily consist of relatively young adults [115]. Acute infection accounts for approximately 60% of hospital admissions among drug abusers and IE is responsible of 5–15% of these episodes [116]. The presence of IE in a drug addict is difficult to predict, especially from history and physical examination findings alone [117, 118]. More than 60% of IV drug abusers with IE do not have an underlying preexisting valvular disease [119]. Although cocaine use by an intravenous drug abuser should raise the suspicion of IE infection [120], the most credible predictors of IE in febrile intravenous drug users are visualization of vegetations by echocardiography and the presence of embolic phenomena [118]. Up to 13% of cases of IV drug abusers with febrile episodes have an echocardiographically demonstrated IE [118]. Although left-sided native valve endocarditis may be present in this group of patients, the tricuspid valve is more commonly affected in intravenous drug users [121, 122]. Only two-third of patients with proven IE diagnostic presented with heart murmurs on admission [116]. The frequency of valvular involvement is tricuspid alone or in combination with other valves, 52.2%; aortic

http://dx.doi.org/10.5772/65030

alone, 18.5%; mitral alone 10.8%; and mitral and aortic combined, 12.5% [123]. Most of these patients are young (20–40 years old), and men are more commonly affected than women with a ratio of 4:1–6:1. Approximately 66% of the patients have extravalvular compromise which may help in the diagnosis [124–126]. Although there are studies reporting infection rate reductions (such as HIV, hepatitis, or abscess) with the implementation of a needle-exchange program [127, 128], to date, there are no conclusive evidence showing reduction in IE among this special group.

3. Conclusions

Much work remains to be completed. IE is a complex and challenging pathology with a high mortality rate despite current advancements in health care. Even though diagnostic and therapeutic modalities have progressed since the "rheumatic fever" era, there is still a concern in developing countries where rheumatic fever represents a major cause of IE and access to appropriate health care is not possible in large areas. Curiously, the changing epidemiology of IE depict us a disease that used to affect young patients, native valves, and had *Streptococci* as the main pathogen, to a disease that affect mainly older people with prosthetic valves implanted and *S. aureus* as the main pathogen. These changes occur alongside a better survival in older people but also with several comorbidities accompanying these patients. Imaging modalities such as echocardiography had greatly helped in the diagnosis of IE; the role of advanced imaging had yet to be clinically evaluated in a day-to-day basis. Chronic and immunosuppressive diseases play a major role as predisposing factors to develop IE. IV drug users comprise other group of patients severely affected by the disease. Adequate clinical analysis and high suspicion are necessary to help these "risk" patients and provide the right tools (multidisciplinary team) to detect and treat this limiting and deadly condition.

Author details

Fabian Andres Giraldo Vallejo

Address all correspondence to: fabiangiraldomd@gmail.com

Instituto del Corazón de Bucaramanga, Bucaramanga, Colombia

References

[1] Lerner PI, Weinstein L. Infective endocarditis in the antibiotic era. N Engl J Med. 1966;274(7):388–93 concl.

[2] Von Reyn CF, Levy BS, Arbeit RD, Friedland G, Crumpacker CS. Infective endocarditis: an analysis based on strict case definitions. Ann Intern Med. 1981;94(4 pt 1):505–18.

[3] Durack DT, Lukes AS, Bright DK. New criteria for diagnosis of infective endocarditis: utilization of specific echocardiographic findings. Duke Endocarditis Service. Am J Med. 1994;96(3):200–9.

[4] Li JS, Sexton DJ, Mick N, Nettles R, Fowler VG, Ryan T, et al. Proposed modifications to the Duke criteria for the diagnosis of infective endocarditis. Clin Infect Dis Off Publ Infect Dis Soc Am. 2000;30(4):633–8.

[5] Evangelista A. Echocardiography in infective endocarditis. Heart. 2004;90(6):614–7.

[6] Greaves K. Clinical criteria and the appropriate use of transthoracic echocardiography for the exclusion of infective endocarditis. Heart. 2003;89(3):273–5.

[7] Vieira MLC. Repeated echocardiographic examinations of patients with suspected infective endocarditis. Heart. 2004;90(9):1020–4.

[8] Prendergast BD. The changing face of infective endocarditis. Heart Br Card Soc. 2006;92(7):879–85.

[9] Murdoch DR. Clinical presentation, etiology, and outcome of infective endocarditis in the 21st century: the International Collaboration on Endocarditis–Prospective Cohort Study. Arch Intern Med. 2009;169(5):463.

[10] Selton-Suty C, Celard M, Le Moing V, Doco-Lecompte T, Chirouze C, Iung B, et al. Preeminence of *Staphylococcus aureus* in infective endocarditis: a 1-year population-based survey. Clin Infect Dis. 2012;54(9):1230–9.

[11] Allegranzi B, Nejad SB, Combescure C, Graafmans W, Attar H, Donaldson L, et al. Burden of endemic health-care-associated infection in developing countries: systematic review and meta-analysis. The Lancet. 2011;377(9761):228–41.

[12] Moreillon P, Que Y-A. Infective endocarditis. The Lancet. 2004;363(9403):139–49.

[13] de Sa DDC, Tleyjeh IM, Anavekar NS, Schultz JC, Thomas JM, Lahr BD, et al. Epidemiological trends of infective endocarditis: a population-based study in Olmsted County, Minnesota. Mayo Clin Proc. 2010;85(5):422–6.

[14] Tleyjeh IM, Abdel-Latif A, Rahbi H, Scott CG, Bailey KR, Steckelberg JM, et al. A systematic review of population-based studies of infective endocarditis. Chest. 2007;132(3):1025–35.

[15] Hasbun R, Vikram HR, Barakat LA, Buenconsejo J, Quagliarello VJ. Complicated left-sided native valve endocarditis in adults: risk classification for mortality. JAMA. 2003;289(15):1933–40.

[16] Chirouze C, Cabell CH, Fowler VG, Khayat N, Olaison L, Miro JM, et al. Prognostic factors in 61 cases of *Staphylococcus aureus* prosthetic valve infective endocarditis from

the International Collaboration on Endocarditis merged database. Clin Infect Dis Off Publ Infect Dis Soc Am. 2004;38(9):1323–7.

[17] Endorsed by the European Society of Clinical Microbiology and Infectious Diseases (ESCMID) and by the International Society of Chemotherapy (ISC) for Infection and Cancer, Authors/Task Force Members, Habib G, Hoen B, Tornos P, Thuny F, et al. Guidelines on the prevention, diagnosis, and treatment of infective endocarditis (new version 2009): The Task Force on the Prevention, Diagnosis, and Treatment of Infective Endocarditis of the European Society of Cardiology (ESC). Eur Heart J. 2009;30(19): 2369–413.

[18] Nishimura RA, Otto CM, Bonow RO, Carabello BA, Erwin JP, Guyton RA, et al. 2014 AHA/ACC guideline for the management of patients with valvular heart disease: a report of the American College of Cardiology/American Heart Association Task Force on Practice Guidelines. Circulation. 2014;129(23):e521–643.

[19] Hoen B, Alla F, Selton-Suty C, Béguinot I, Bouvet A, Briançon S, et al. Changing profile of infective endocarditis: results of a 1-year survey in France. JAMA. 2002;288(1):75–81.

[20] Letaief A, Boughzala E, Kaabia N, Ernez S, Abid F, Ben Chaabane T, et al. Epidemiology of infective endocarditis in Tunisia: a 10-year multicenter retrospective study. Int J Infect Dis IJID Off Publ Int Soc Infect Dis. 2007;11(5):430–3.

[21] Hill EE, Herijgers P, Claus P, Vanderschueren S, Herregods M-C, Peetermans WE. Infective endocarditis: changing epidemiology and predictors of 6-month mortality: a prospective cohort study. Eur Heart J. 2007;28(2):196–203.

[22] Cabell CH, Jollis JG, Peterson GE, Corey GR, Anderson DJ, Sexton DJ, et al. Changing patient characteristics and the effect on mortality in endocarditis. Arch Intern Med. 2002;162(1):90–4.

[23] Fowler VG, Miro JM, Hoen B, Cabell CH, Abrutyn E, Rubinstein E, et al. *Staphylococcus aureus* endocarditis: a consequence of medical progress. JAMA. 2005;293(24):3012–21.

[24] Lopez J, Revilla A, Vilacosta I, Sevilla T, Villacorta E, Sarria C, et al. Age-dependent profile of left-sided infective endocarditis: a 3-center experience. Circulation. 2010;121(7):892–7.

[25] Durante-Mangoni E. Current features of infective endocarditis in elderly patients: results of the International Collaboration on Endocarditis Prospective Cohort Study. Arch Intern Med. 2008;168(19):2095.

[26] Steckelberg JM, Melton LJ, Ilstrup DM, Rouse MS, Wilson WR. Influence of referral bias on the apparent clinical spectrum of infective endocarditis. Am J Med. 1990;88(6):582–8.

[27] Tleyjeh IM, Steckelberg JM, Murad HS, Anavekar NS, Ghomrawi HMK, Mirzoyev Z, et al. Temporal trends in infective endocarditis: a population-based study in Olmsted County, Minnesota. JAMA. 2005;293(24):3022–8.

[28] King JW, Nguyen VQ, Conrad SA. Results of a prospective statewide reporting system for infective endocarditis. Am J Med Sci. 1988;295(6):517–27.

[29] Delahaye F, Goulet V, Lacassin F, Ecochard R, Selton-Suty C, Hoen B, et al. Characteristics of infective endocarditis in France in 1991. A 1-year survey. Eur Heart J. 1995;16(3): 394–401.

[30] SHULMAN ST. Infective endocarditis: 1986. Pediatr Infect Dis J [Internet]. 1986;5(6). Available from: http://journals.lww.com/pidj/Fulltext/1986/11000/Infective_endocarditis__1986_.18.aspx.

[31] Berlin JA, Abrutyn E, Strom BL, Kinman JL, Levison ME, Korzeniowski OM, et al. Incidence of infective endocarditis in the Delaware Valley, 1988-1990. Am J Cardiol. 1995;76(12):933–6.

[32] Federspiel JJ. Increasing US rates of endocarditis with *Staphylococcus aureus*: 1999-2008. Arch Intern Med. 2012;172(4):363.

[33] Normand J, Bozio A, Etienne J, Sassolas F, Le Bris H. Changing patterns and prognosis of infective endocarditis in childhood. Eur Heart J. 1995;16(Suppl B):28–31.

[34] Carapetis JR, Steer AC, Mulholland EK, Weber M. The global burden of group A *Streptococcal* diseases. Lancet Infect Dis. 2005;5(11):685–94.

[35] Marijon E, Ou P, Celermajer DS, Ferreira B, Mocumbi AO, Jani D, et al. Prevalence of rheumatic heart disease detected by echocardiographic screening. N Engl J Med. 2007;357(5):470–6.

[36] Thayer WS. Studies on bacterial (infective) endocarditis. Johns Hopkins Hosp Rep. 1926;22(1):1–8.

[37] Slipczuk L, Codolosa JN, Davila CD, Romero-Corral A, Yun J, Pressman GS, et al. Infective endocarditis epidemiology over five decades: a systematic review. Schlievert PM, editor. PLoS ONE. 2013;8(12):e82665.

[38] Fernández-Guerrero ML, Verdejo C, Azofra J, de Górgolas M. Hospital-acquired infectious endocarditis not associated with cardiac surgery: an emerging problem. Clin Infect Dis Off Publ Infect Dis Soc Am. 1995;20(1):16–23.

[39] Gouëllo JP, Asfar P, Brenet O, Kouatchet A, Berthelot G, Alquier P. Nosocomial endocarditis in the intensive care unit: an analysis of 22 cases. Crit Care Med. 2000;28(2): 377–82.

[40] Benito N, Miró JM, de Lazzari E, Cabell CH, del Río A, Altclas J, et al. Health care-associated native valve endocarditis: importance of non-nosocomial acquisition. Ann Intern Med. 2009;150(9):586–94.

[41] Martín-Dávila P, Fortún J, Navas E, Cobo J, Jiménez-Mena M, Moya JL, et al. Nosocomial endocarditis in a tertiary hospital: an increasing trend in native valve cases. Chest. 2005;128(2):772–9.

[42] Karchmer AW, Longworth DL. Infections of intracardiac devices. Cardiol Clin. 2003;21(2):253–71, vii.

[43] Rivas P, Alonso J, Moya J, de Górgolas M, Martinell J, Fernández Guerrero ML. The impact of hospital-acquired infections on the microbial etiology and prognosis of late-onset prosthetic valve endocarditis. Chest. 2005;128(2):764–71.

[44] Come PC. Infective endocarditis: current perspectives. Compr Ther. 1982;8(7):57–70.

[45] Kamalakannan D, Pai RM, Johnson LB, Gardin JM, Saravolatz LD. Epidemiology and clinical outcomes of infective endocarditis in hemodialysis patients. Ann Thorac Surg. 2007;83(6):2081–6.

[46] Hoen B. Infective endocarditis: a frequent disease in dialysis patients. Nephrol Dial Transplant Off Publ Eur Dial Transpl Assoc Eur Ren Assoc. 2004;19(6):1360–2.

[47] Fowler VG, Sanders LL, Kong LK, McClelland RS, Gottlieb GS, Li J, et al. Infective endocarditis due to *Staphylococcus aureus*: 59 prospectively identified cases with follow-up. Clin Infect Dis Off Publ Infect Dis Soc Am. 1999;28(1):106–14.

[48] Chang F-Y, MacDonald BB, Peacock JE, Musher DM, Triplett P, Mylotte JM, et al. A prospective multicenter study of *Staphylococcus aureus* bacteremia: incidence of endocarditis, risk factors for mortality, and clinical impact of methicillin resistance. Medicine (Baltimore). 2003;82(5):322–32.

[49] Schell HM. The immunocompromised host and risk for cardiovascular infection. J Cardiovasc Nurs. 1999;13(2):31–48.

[50] Pulvirenti JJ, Kerns E, Benson C, Lisowski J, Demarais P, Weinstein RA. Infective endocarditis in injection drug users: importance of human immunodeficiency virus serostatus and degree of immunosuppression. Clin Infect Dis Off Publ Infect Dis Soc Am. 1996;22(1):40–5.

[51] Ribera E, Miró JM, Cortés E, Cruceta A, Merce J, Marco F, et al. Influence of human immunodeficiency virus 1 infection and degree of immunosuppression in the clinical characteristics and outcome of infective endocarditis in intravenous drug users. Arch Intern Med. 1998;158(18):2043–50.

[52] Fisher SD LS. Cardiovascular abnormalities in HIV-infected individuals. In: Braunwald E, editor. Heart disease: a textbook of cardiovascular medicine. 6th ed. Philadelphia: Saunders; 2001. pp. 2211–21.

[53] Wang A, Athan E, Pappas PA, Fowler VG, Olaison L, Paré C, et al. Contemporary clinical profile and outcome of prosthetic valve endocarditis. JAMA. 2007;297(12):1354–61.

[54] Habib G, Tribouilloy C, Thuny F, Giorgi R, Brahim A, Amazouz M, et al. Prosthetic valve endocarditis: who needs surgery? A multicentre study of 104 cases. Heart Br Card Soc. 2005;91(7):954–9.

[55] Hyde JA, Darouiche RO, Costerton JW. Strategies for prophylaxis against prosthetic valve endocarditis: a review article. J Heart Valve Dis. 1998;7(3):316–26.

[56] Calderwood SB, Swinski LA, Waternaux CM, Karchmer AW, Buckley MJ. Risk factors for the development of prosthetic valve endocarditis. Circulation. 1985;72(1):31–7.

[57] Glower DD, Landolfo KP, Cheruvu S, Cen YY, Harrison JK, Bashore TM, et al. Determinants of 15-year outcome with 1,119 standard Carpentier-Edwards porcine valves. Ann Thorac Surg. 1998;66(6 Suppl):S44–8.

[58] Ivert TS, Dismukes WE, Cobbs CG, Blackstone EH, Kirklin JW, Bergdahl LA. Prosthetic valve endocarditis. Circulation. 1984;69(2):223–32.

[59] Murashita T. Surgical results for active endocarditis with prosthetic valve replacement: impact of culture-negative endocarditis on early and late outcomes. Eur J Cardiothorac Surg. 2004;26(6):1104–11.

[60] Tornos P. Infective endocarditis in Europe: lessons from the Euro heart survey. Heart. 2005;91(5):571–5.

[61] Romano G, Carozza A, Della Corte A, De Santo LS, Amarelli C, Torella M, et al. Native versus primary prosthetic valve endocarditis: comparison of clinical features and long-term outcome in 353 patients. J Heart Valve Dis. 2004;13(2):200–8; discussion 208–9.

[62] Sohail MR, Martin KR, Wilson WR, Baddour LM, Harmsen WS, Steckelberg JM. Medical versus surgical management of *Staphylococcus aureus* prosthetic valve endocarditis. Am J Med. 2006;119(2):147–54.

[63] Piper C. Valve disease: prosthetic valve endocarditis. Heart. 2001;85(5):590–3.

[64] Arvay A, Lengyel M. Incidence and risk factors of prosthetic valve endocarditis. Eur J Cardio-Thorac Surg Off J Eur Assoc Cardio-Thorac Surg. 1988;2(5):340–6.

[65] Hammermeister K, Sethi GK, Henderson WG, Grover FL, Oprian C, Rahimtoola SH. Outcomes 15 years after valve replacement with a mechanical versus a bioprosthetic valve: final report of the Veterans Affairs randomized trial. J Am Coll Cardiol. 2000;36(4):1152–8.

[66] Agnihotri A, Mcgiffin D, Galbraith A, Obrien M. The prevalence of infective endocarditis after aortic valve replacement. J Thorac Cardiovasc Surg. 1995;110(6):1708–24.

[67] Vongpatanasin W, Hillis LD, Lange RA. Prosthetic heart valves. N Engl J Med. 1996;335(6):407–16.

[68] Sidhu P, O'Kane H, Ali N, Gladstone DJ, Sarsam MA, Campalani G, et al. Mechanical or bioprosthetic valves in the elderly: a 20-year comparison. Ann Thorac Surg. 2001;71(5 Suppl):S257–60.

[69] Tornos P, Almirante B, Olona M, Permanyer G, González T, Carballo J, et al. Clinical outcome and long-term prognosis of late prosthetic valve endocarditis: a 20-year experience. Clin Infect Dis Off Publ Infect Dis Soc Am. 1997;24(3):381–6.

[70] Wilson WR, Jaumin PM, Danielson GK, Giuliani ER, Washington JA II, Geraci JE. Prosthetic valve endocarditis. Ann Intern Med. 1975;82(6):751–6.

[71] López J, Revilla A, Vilacosta I, Villacorta E, González-Juanatey C, Gómez I, et al. Definition, clinical profile, microbiological spectrum, and prognostic factors of early-onset prosthetic valve endocarditis. Eur Heart J. 2007;28(6):760–5.

[72] Latib A, Naim C, De Bonis M, Sinning JM, Maisano F, Barbanti M, et al. TAVR-associated prosthetic valve infective endocarditis. J Am Coll Cardiol. 2014;64(20):2176–8.

[73] Baddour LM, Cha Y-M, Wilson WR. Infections of cardiovascular implantable electronic devices. N Engl J Med. 2012;367(9):842–9.

[74] Sohail MR. Mortality and cost associated with cardiovascular implantable electronic device infections. Arch Intern Med. 2011;171(20):1821.

[75] Greenspon AJ, Patel JD, Lau E, Ochoa JA, Frisch DR, Ho RT, et al. 16-Year Trends in the infection burden for pacemakers and implantable cardioverter-defibrillators in the United States. J Am Coll Cardiol. 2011;58(10):1001–6.

[76] Sohail MR, Uslan DZ, Khan AH, Friedman PA, Hayes DL, Wilson WR, et al. Management and outcome of permanent pacemaker and implantable cardioverter-defibrillator infections. J Am Coll Cardiol. 2007;49(18):1851–9.

[77] Lai KK, Fontecchio SA. Infections associated with implantable cardioverter defibrillators placed transvenously and via thoracotomies: epidemiology, infection control, and management. Clin Infect Dis Off Publ Infect Dis Soc Am. 1998;27(2):265–9.

[78] Mela T, McGovern BA, Garan H, Vlahakes GJ, Torchiana DF, Ruskin J, et al. Long-term infection rates associated with the pectoral versus abdominal approach to cardioverter-defibrillator implants. Am J Cardiol. 2001;88(7):750–3.

[79] Voigt A, Shalaby A, Saba S. Rising rates of cardiac rhythm management device infections in the United States: 1996 through 2003. J Am Coll Cardiol. 2006;48(3):590–1.

[80] Sohail MR, Uslan DZ, Khan AH, Friedman PA, Hayes DL, Wilson WR, et al. Risk factor analysis of permanent pacemaker infection. Clin Infect Dis Off Publ Infect Dis Soc Am. 2007;45(2):166–73.

[81] Uslan DZ, Sohail MR, St Sauver JL, Friedman PA, Hayes DL, Stoner SM, et al. Permanent pacemaker and implantable cardioverter defibrillator infection: a population-based study. Arch Intern Med. 2007;167(7):669–75.

[82] Topkara VK, Kondareddy S, Malik F, Wang I-W, Mann DL, Ewald GA, et al. Infectious complications in patients with left ventricular assist device: etiology and outcomes in the continuous-flow era. Ann Thorac Surg. 2010;90(4):1270–7.

[83] Hravnak M, George E, Kormos RL. Management of chronic left ventricular assist device percutaneous lead insertion sites. J Heart Lung Transplant Off Publ Int Soc Heart Transplant. 1993;12(5):856–63.

[84] Baddour LM. Nonvalvular cardiovascular device-related infections. Circulation. 2003;108(16):2015–31.

[85] Allen HD, Beekman RH, Garson A, Hijazi ZM, Mullins C, O'Laughlin MP, et al. Pediatric therapeutic cardiac catheterization: a statement for healthcare professionals from the Council on Cardiovascular Disease in the Young, American Heart Association. Circulation. 1998;97(6):609–25.

[86] Rao PS, Sideris EB, Hausdorf G, Rey C, Lloyd TR, Beekman RH, et al. International experience with secundum atrial septal defect occlusion by the buttoned device. Am Heart J. 1994;128(5):1022–35.

[87] Pihkala J, Nykanen D, Freedom RM, Benson LN. Interventional cardiac catheterization. Pediatr Clin North Am. 1999;46(2):441–64.

[88] Zamora R, Rao PS, Lloyd TR, Beekman RH, Sideris EB. Intermediate-term results of Phase I Food and Drug Administration Trials of buttoned device occlusion of secundum atrial septal defects. J Am Coll Cardiol. 1998;31(3):674–6.

[89] Goldstein JA, Beardslee MA, Xu H, Sundt TM, Lasala JM. Infective endocarditis resulting from CardioSEAL closure of a patent foramen ovale. Catheter Cardiovasc Interv Off J Soc Card Angiogr Interv. 2002;55(2):217–20; discussion 221.

[90] Bullock AM, Menahem S, Wilkinson JL. Infective endocarditis on an occluder closing an atrial septal defect. Cardiol Young. 1999;9(1):65–7.

[91] Johnson DH, Rosenthal A, Nadas AS. A forty-year review of bacterial endocarditis in infancy and childhood. Circulation. 1975;51(4):581–8.

[92] Van Hare GF, Ben-Shachar G, Liebman J, Boxerbaum B, Riemenschneider TA. Infective endocarditis in infants and children during the past 10 years: a decade of change. Am Heart J. 1984;107(6):1235–40.

[93] Pasquali SK, He X, Mohamad Z, McCrindle BW, Newburger JW, Li JS, et al. Trends in endocarditis hospitalizations at US children's hospitals: impact of the 2007 American Heart Association Antibiotic Prophylaxis Guidelines. Am Heart J. 2012;163(5):894–9.

[94] Rushani D, Kaufman JS, Ionescu-Ittu R, Mackie AS, Pilote L, Therrien J, et al. Infective endocarditis in children with congenital heart disease: cumulative incidence and predictors. Circulation. 2013;128(13):1412–9.

[95] Day MD, Gauvreau K, Shulman S, Newburger JW. Characteristics of children hospitalized with infective endocarditis. Circulation. 2009;119(6):865–70.

[96] Stull TL LJ. Endocarditis in children. In: Kaye D, editor. Infective endocarditis. 2nd ed. New York, NY: Raven Press; pp. 313–27.

[97] Rosenthal LB, Feja KN, Levasseur SM, Alba LR, Gersony W, Saiman L. The changing epidemiology of pediatric endocarditis at a children's hospital over seven decades. Pediatr Cardiol. 2010;31(6):813–20.

[98] Saiman L, Prince A, Gersony WM. Pediatric infective endocarditis in the modern era. J Pediatr. 1993;122(6):847–53.

[99] Morris CD, Reller MD, Menashe VD. Thirty-year incidence of infective endocarditis after surgery for congenital heart defect. JAMA. 1998;279(8):599–603.

[100] Stockheim JA, Chadwick EG, Kessler S, Amer M, Abdel-Haq N, Dajani AS, et al. Are the Duke criteria superior to the Beth Israel criteria for the diagnosis of infective endocarditis in children? Clin Infect Dis Off Publ Infect Dis Soc Am. 1998;27(6):1451–6.

[101] Valente AM. Frequency of infective endocarditis among infants and children with *Staphylococcus aureus* bacteremia. PEDIATRICS [Internet]. 2004 December 15 [cited 2016 June 13]; Available from: http://pediatrics.aappublications.org/cgi/doi/10.1542/peds.2004-1152.

[102] Tribouilloy C, Rusinaru D, Sorel C, Thuny F, Casalta J-P, Riberi A, et al. Clinical characteristics and outcome of infective endocarditis in adults with bicuspid aortic valves: a multicentre observational study. Heart. 2010;96(21):1723–9.

[103] McKinsey DS, Ratts TE, Bisno AL. Underlying cardiac lesions in adults with infective endocarditis. The changing spectrum. Am J Med. 1987;82(4):681–8.

[104] Fulkerson PK, Beaver BM, Auseon JC, Graber HL. Calcification of the mitral annulus: etiology, clinical associations, complications and therapy. Am J Med. 1979;66(6):967–77.

[105] Chagnac A, Rudniki C, Loebel H, Zahavi I. Infectious endocarditis in idiopathic hypertrophic subaortic stenosis: report of three cases and review of the literature. Chest. 1982;81(3):346–9.

[106] Corrigall D, Bolen J, Hancock EW, Popp RL. Mitral valve prolapse and infective endocarditis. Am J Med. 1977;63(2):215–22.

[107] Yang L, Gu X, Zhang X. [Mitral valve prolapse and infective endocarditis]. Zhonghua Nei Ke Za Zhi. 1997;36(12):802–4.

[108] Jeresaty RM. Mitral valve prolapse–Click syndrome. Prog Cardiovasc Dis. 1973;15(6):623–52.

[109] Schutte JE, Gaffney FA, Blend L, Blomqvist CG. Distinctive anthropometric characteristics of women with mitral valve prolapse. Am J Med. 1981;71(4):533–8.

[110] Devereux RB, Kramer-Fox R, Kligfield P. Mitral valve prolapse: causes, clinical manifestations, and management. Ann Intern Med. 1989;111(4):305–17.

[111] Clemens JD, Horwitz RI, Jaffe CC, Feinstein AR, Stanton BF. A controlled evaluation of the risk of bacterial endocarditis in persons with mitral-valve prolapse. N Engl J Med. 1982;307(13):776–81.

[112] Nolan CM, Kane JJ, Grunow WA. Infective endocarditis and mitral prolapse: a comparison with other types of endocarditis. Arch Intern Med. 1981;141(4):447–50.

[113] Sande, M. A. LB, Mills J. CIH. Endocarditis in intravenous drug users. In: Kaye D, editor. Infective endocarditis. 2nd ed. New York, NY: Raven Press; 1992. pp. 345–9.

[114] Weinstein L, Brusch JL, editors. In: Infective endocarditis. New York, NY: Oxford University Press; 1996. pp. 194–209.

[115] Wilson LE, Thomas DL, Astemborski J, Freedman TL, Vlahov D. Prospective study of infective endocarditis among injection drug users. J Infect Dis. 2002;185(12):1761–6.

[116] Levine DP, Crane LR, Zervos MJ. Bacteremia in narcotic addicts at the Detroit Medical Center. II. Infectious endocarditis: a prospective comparative study. Rev Infect Dis. 1986;8(3):374–96.

[117] Marantz PR, Linzer M, Feiner CJ, Feinstein SA, Kozin AM, Friedland GH. Inability to predict diagnosis in febrile intravenous drug abusers. Ann Intern Med. 1987;106(6):823–8.

[118] Weisse AB, Heller DR, Schimenti RJ, Montgomery RL, Kapila R. The febrile parenteral drug user: a prospective study in 121 patients. Am J Med. 1993;94(3):274–80.

[119] Miró JM, Moreno A, Mestres CA. Infective endocarditis in intravenous drug abusers. Curr Infect Dis Rep. 2003;5(4):307–16.

[120] Chambers HF, Morris DL, Täuber MG, Modin G. Cocaine use and the risk for endocarditis in intravenous drug users. Ann Intern Med. 1987;106(6):833–6.

[121] Moss R, Munt B. Injection drug use and right sided endocarditis. Heart Br Card Soc. 2003;89(5):577–81.

[122] Mathew J, Addai T, Anand A, Morrobel A, Maheshwari P, Freels S. Clinical features, site of involvement, bacteriologic findings, and outcome of infective endocarditis in intravenous drug users. Arch Intern Med. 1995;155(15):1641–8.

[123] Carozza A, De Santo LS, Romano G, Della Corte A, Ursomando F, Scardone M, et al. Infective endocarditis in intravenous drug abusers: patterns of presentation and long-term outcomes of surgical treatment. J Heart Valve Dis. 2006;15(1):125–31.

[124] Chambers HF, Korzeniowski OM, Sande MA. *Staphylococcus aureus* endocarditis: clinical manifestations in addicts and nonaddicts. Medicine (Baltimore). 1983;62(3): 170–7.

[125] Sklaver AR, Hoffman TA, Greenman RL. *Staphylococcal* endocarditis in addicts. South Med J. 1978;71(6):638–43.

[126] Thadepalli H, Francis CK. Diagnostic clues in metastatic lesions of endocarditis in addicts. West J Med. 1978;128(1):1–5.

[127] Braine N, Jarlais DCD, Ahmad S, Purchase D, Turner C. Long-term effects of syringe exchange on risk behavior and HIV prevention. AIDS Educ Prev. 2004;16(3):264–75.

[128] Vlahov D, Junge B. The role of needle exchange programs in HIV prevention. Public Health Rep Wash DC 1974. 1998;113(Suppl 1):75–80.

Section 3

Diagnosis

Chapter 4

Advanced Echocardiography for the Diagnosis and Management of Infective Endocarditis

John F. Sedgwick and Gregory M. Scalia

Additional information is available at the end of the chapter

http://dx.doi.org/10.5772/64800

Abstract

Echocardiography is fundamental for the management of infective endocarditis (IE) across all stages of the illness including diagnosis, surveillance during medical therapy, identification of prognostic markers, planning perioperative intervention, postoperative assessment, and follow-up after completion of definitive therapy. Modern era echocardiography (echo) offers outstanding temporal and spatial image resolution, providing the opportunity for early diagnosis of this life-threatening infection. Emerging imaging modalities, such as real-time three-dimensional (3D) echocardiography, offer a novel way of readily visualizing the extent of intracardiac infection and the relationship of pathology to adjacent cardiac structures, well before surgical intervention, without radiation exposure or significant risk to the patient. Echocardiography can have a positive impact on the management of every stage of this disease, with the opportunity to improve outcomes.

Keywords: transthoracic echocardiography, transesophageal echocardiography, 3D echocardiography, infective endocarditis, cardiac device-related endocarditis, left-sided endocarditis, right-sided endocarditis, native valve infection, prosthetic valve infection, vegetation, abscess, diagnosis, congenital heart disease, diagnostic accuracy, sensitivity, specificity, management, surgery, cardiac imaging, intracardiac ultrasound

1. Introduction

Echocardiography is fundamental to the diagnosis, risk stratification, management, and follow-up of patients with IE [1]. Modern era transthoracic echocardiography (TTE) and transesophageal echocardiography (TEE) enable cardiac anatomy, pathology, and physiology to be assessed in real time. Echocardiography is a readily available, portable imaging modality that uses the properties of reflected ultrasound waves to construct high-quality two-dimensional (2D) and three-dimensional (3D) images of the heart without radiation exposure. Echocardiography should be utilized at the first opportunity when IE is suspected, to provide an early diagnosis and facilitate important management decisions. However, echocardiographic findings should always be interpreted in their clinical context to maximize diagnostic utility.

This chapter will outline the role echocardiography in the management of IE. In addition, the history of cardiac ultrasound, its diagnostic accuracy, limitations, and emerging technologies such as 3D imaging will be reviewed. Finally, there is a section on imaging protocols and quality control to provide guidance to echocardiography laboratories wishing to pursue excellence in the field.

2. Diagnosis

The modified Duke criteria [2] is used to categorize endocarditis as definite, possible or rejected based on clinical, microbiological, echocardiographic, and pathological findings. Blood cultures and echocardiography are the two key criteria for IE. The modified Duke criteria [2] has an overall sensitivity of ~80–90%, and specificity >90% for diagnosis of IE when compared to pathological diagnosis; however, it is less reliable for identification of prosthetic valve endocarditis (PVE) with sensitivity ~70–80% [3–7]. Transesophageal echocardiography has been shown to improve the diagnostic accuracy of the Duke criteria for definite IE when compared with TTE imaging [8].

A high-clinical suspicion for IE should be adopted especially when fever is present in patients with a prosthetic valve or device, new murmur or heart block, underlying valvular disease or congenital heart disease (CHD), embolism, immunosuppression, previous IE, or intravenous drug abuse (IVDA). It is imperative for early blood cultures be collected prior to antibiotic therapy and urgent echocardiography performed.

2.1. Major Duke echocardiographic findings

The three major echocardiographic findings as defined by the modified Duke criteria [2] suggesting direct evidence of endocardial involvement are vegetation, abscess, and new partial dehiscence of a prosthetic valve.

Vegetation is seen as a high frequency independently oscillating mass typically located on the low-pressure side of cardiac valves, in particular the atrial aspect of the atrioventricular (mitral and tricuspid) valves and the outflow tract side of the semilunar (aortic and pulmonary) valves (**Figure 1**). Less often, vegetations can be sessile with little or no mobility or have mixed sessile and mobile components.

Vegetations are commonly attached along the leaflet coaptation zone, although it can be located anywhere on the valve leaflet, annulus, and subvalvular apparatus. They are also frequently found in the path of abnormal turbulent blood flow ('jet lesion') arising from

http://dx.doi.org/10.5772/64800

valvular regurgitation, a shunt or may spread to adjacent structures by direct contact ('kissing lesion'). Vegetations may also be attached to the endocardial surface lining the heart chambers (mural) or blood vessels (intraluminal). With an aging population and increased cardiac interventions, vegetations involving prosthetic valves, pacing leads, and other non-biological intracardiac materials are becoming more prevalent (**Figure 2**).

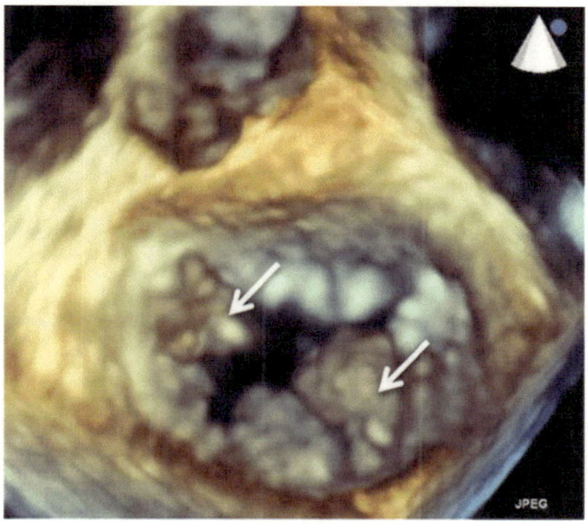

Figure 1. 3D TEE en-face view of mitral valve demonstrating multiple vegetations (arrows).

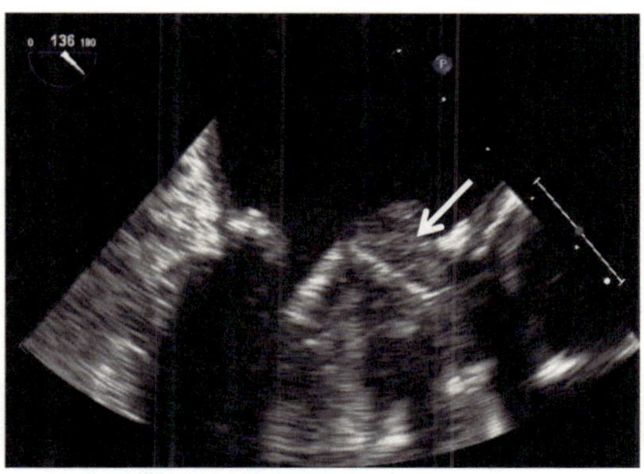

Figure 2. TEE mitral valve with large vegetation causing a 'stuck' anterior mechanical occluder (arrow).

A vegetation has a similar 'gray scale' ultrasound reflectance (echogenicity) to normal myocardium. Chronic 'healed' vegetations, however, often become partly calcified and therefore appear more echogenic when compared to surrounding structures. Vegetations usually have a soft 'shaggy' irregular inhomogeneous appearance on echocardiography helping to differentiate them from simple degenerative valvular tissue strands such as Lambl's excrescences, which tend to be very thin linear structures (**Figure 3**). Vegetations may reduce in size with treatment, embolize, or remain unchanged.

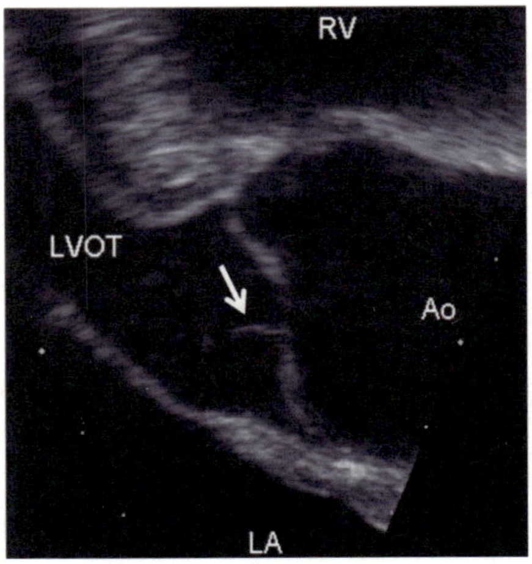

Figure 3. TEE demonstrating the common finding of a degenerative 'Lambl's excrescence' attached to the LVOT aspect (arrow) of the aortic valve.

Differential diagnoses for such masses include fibrin and thrombus, which are frequently extremely difficult, if not impossible to distinguish from vegetations on ultrasound imaging. Other findings, such as pannus and tumors, often have a characteristically distinct appearance from vegetations, albeit subtle, and therefore, it is not always possible to differentiate from one another. While imaging cannot specifically identify the type of microorganism, the appearance/ complications of a vegetation may suggest infective agents, for example, fungal vegetations tend to grow to a very large size, and staphylococcus is associated with abscess.

A minority of vegetations are noninfective in origin and referred to as nonbacterial thrombotic endocarditis (NBTE). According to one study [9], lesions resembling NBTE vegetations were identified by echocardiography frequently in patients with antiphospholipid syndrome/ Libman–Sacks (63%), myeloproliferative disorders (63%), and solid-organ malignancies (19%). The lesions most often resembled typical vegetations, but also diffuse valve involvement (e.g., **Figure 4**), with a verrucous appearance can occur [9–11].

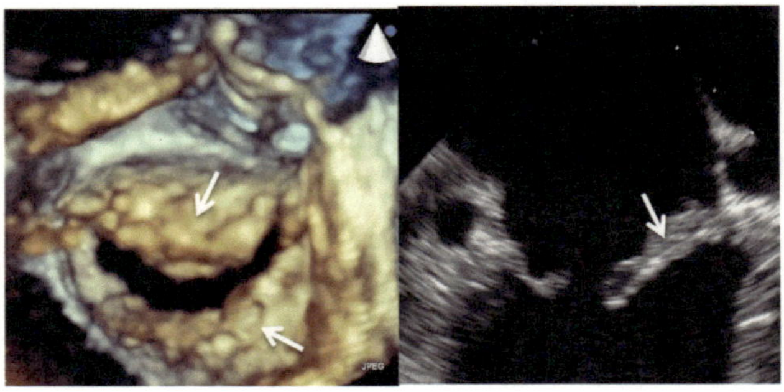

Figure 4. Diffuse, 'verrucous' (arrows) thickening of mitral leaflets in Libman–Sacks endocarditis. Three-dimensional TEE mitral valve (LVOT aspect) and 2D TEE mid esophageal view, mitral valve.

http://dx.doi.org/10.5772/64800

Intracardiac abscesses appear as inhomogeneous echolucent or occasionally echodense regions, involving the periannular tissue or myocardium, comprised of necrotic and purulent material. A developing abscess may present as a region of periannular thickening (≥10 mm) and is referred to as a *phlegmon*. Importantly, there is no color flow on Doppler imaging into an abscess from the vessel lumen or cardiac chamber.

Abscesses are detected in patients undergoing surgery for endocarditis at the aortic annulus in 33–50% of cases, but only 10–20% are located at the mitral annulus [12–14]. Abscesses account for a higher proportion of complications in PVE (**Figure 5**) and often require surgical intervention [12, 15]. Intervalvular extension of the abscess posteriorly to involve the mitral–aortic intervalvular fibrosa (MAIVF) occurs in approximately two-thirds of aortic periannular infections [16]. In the early stages following aortic valve or root surgery, it may be difficult to distinguish normal postoperative periaortic edema and hematoma from an abscess.

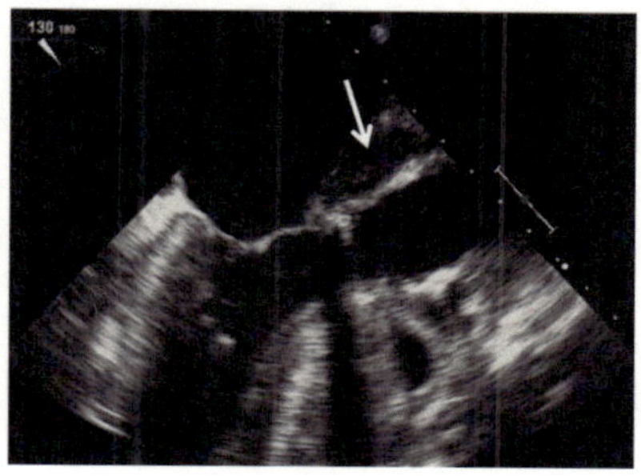

Figure 5. TEE demonstrating posterior periprosthetic aortic abscess (arrow).

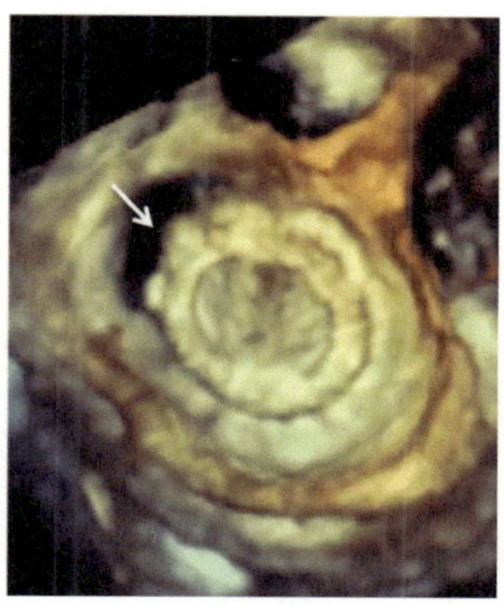

Figure 6. 3D TEE en face of a prosthetic mitral valve with dehiscence at the lateral annulus (arrow).

Mitral annular abscess is often located at the mural annulus, particularly the posterior or lateral annular margin [17], rather than the septal annulus [14]. Mitral annular abscess is more frequently associated with pseudoaneurysm formation and/or fistula than aortic abscess.

Complications include rupture into the coronary sinus, left circumflex artery, or the pericardial space [14]. The presence of mitral annular calcification (MAC), especially caseous calcification, can make diagnosis of annular abscess more challenging due to acoustic shadowing artifact.

New dehiscence of a prosthetic valve occurs when there is disruption of the annular sewing ring due to a breakdown of supporting tissue adjacent to the prosthesis (**Figure 6**). This results in perivalvular regurgitation and may be associated with an abnormal rocking motion. If the area of dehiscence around a bioprosthetic aortic valve is <30%, concordant motion of the valve with the aortic root will occur; however, if >40% of annular area is dehisced, discordant or rocking valvular motion will be present (**Figure 7**) [18].

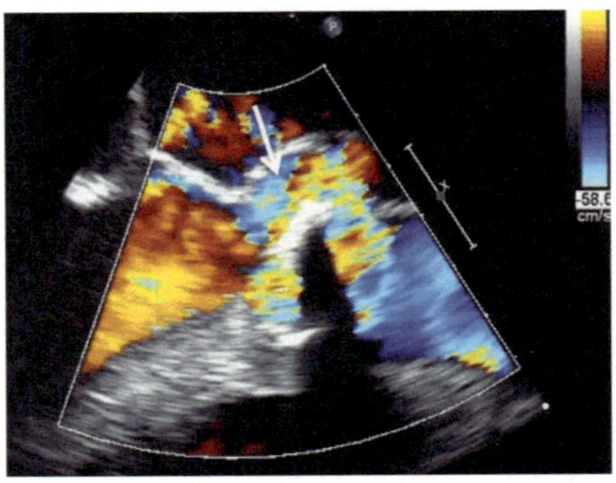

Figure 7. TEE color flow imaging from the 'long-axis' window demonstrating severe periprosthetic aortic valve regurgitation complicating annular dehiscence (arrow). A large region of dehiscence results in a 'rocking' motion of the prosthetic valve.

2.2. Minor Duke echocardiographic findings

Minor echocardiographic findings include but are not limited to perforation, valve aneurysm, fistula, pseudoaneurysm, valve leaflet destruction, and flail leaflet [2].

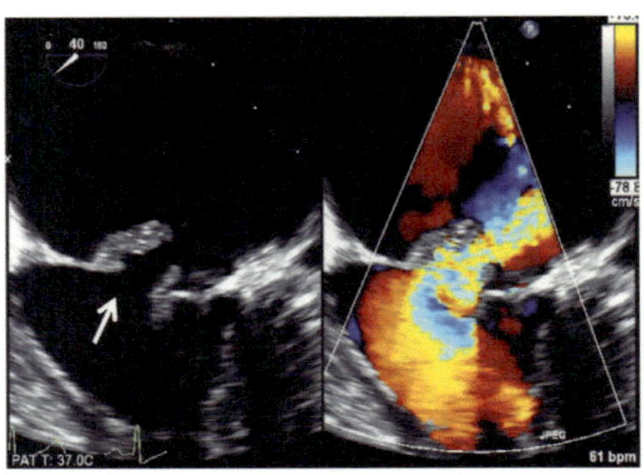

Figure 8. TEE color compare imaging of mitral valve vegetation with perforation (arrow) and severe regurgitation.

http://dx.doi.org/10.5772/64800

The first case report of TEE used to diagnose a perforation was published in 1991 [19]. A perforation is typically a defect through the valvular tissue, separate from the commissures and leaflet margins, well circumscribed and with a 'punched out' appearance on 3D imaging. The finding of a suspected perforation on 2D or 3D echo must be confirmed by demonstrating Doppler color flow traversing the body of the leaflet, typically characterized by flow convergence with a proximal isovelocity surface area (PISA) dome (**Figure 8**).

A valvular aneurysm occurs as a localized bulging sac of the valve leaflet tissue with pulsatile flow seen into the region during systole. The lesion most commonly involves the anterior mitral valve leaflet (AMVL) and usually arises secondary to aortic valve endocarditis [20, 21]. This occurs by either an infected aortic valve regurgitant jet 'seeding' the AMVL or alternatively, from contiguous spread along MAIVF. Localized infection of the mitral leaflet may be followed by valve aneurysm, perforation, and/or leaflet destruction [21].

Cardiac fistula is an uncommon, serious complication, occurring in <1–2.2% [22, 23] of patients with endocarditis and 6–9% of cases when abscess is present [22]. Fistulae often arise from the aortic root or the left ventricular outflow tract [24]. Aortic root fistulas form communications between the aorta and cardiac chambers (aortocavitary) and/or pericardial space (aortopericardial) and often result in hemodynamic compromise. Fistulas can also arise between cardiac chambers [25].

A pseudoaneurysm is defined on echocardiography as an echolucent space communicating with an adjacent cardiac chamber or with the aortic lumen. Blood enters into the cavity under pressure during systole and is seen as pulsatile flow on color Doppler imaging. Pseudoaneurysms frequently arise from the MAIVF with a communication to the left ventricular outflow tract through the narrow 'neck' of the aneurysmal sac [16]. Rupture of a pseudoaneurysm can result in a fistulous connection with the pericardial space, left atrium, or aortic lumen [16, 26].

3. Indications and appropriateness criteria for echocardiography

3.1. American-based guidelines

According to the 2014 ACC/AHA guidelines [27], TTE is indicated in patients with suspected IE to identify vegetations and assess valve hemodynamics, ventricular function, pulmonary pressures, and cardiac complications (class I recommendations). Transesophageal echo is indicated when TTE is nondiagnostic in suspected or known IE, including when intracardiac devices are present and to assess intracardiac complications of IE (class I recommendations). Up to 30% of *Staphylococcus aureus* bacteremia are associated with IE, and therefore, TEE should be strongly considered. In cases where fever defervesced within 72 h and there is a clear extracardiac source (excluding osteomyelitis, spinal involvement, intracardiac device, hemodialysis, structural cardiac disease, prolonged bacteremia, or risk factors), TEE may not be necessary [27].

Another set of independent Guidelines that were published in 2011 by the American College of Cardiology Foundation Quality Strategic Directions Committee Appropriateness Criteria

Working Groups in consultation with other key organizations, developed a scoring system graded from 1 to 9, with 7–9 being an appropriate echo referral, 4–6 uncertain, and 1–3 inappropriate [28]. A summary of the guideline is provided as follows:

3.1.1. Transthoracic imaging

Imaging of native or prosthetic valves is considered most appropriate (grade 9) where endocarditis is clinically suspected and associated with positive blood cultures or a new murmur. In addition, TTE is indicated for reevaluation of IE if any of the following are present as follows: (a) high risk of progressive disease, (b) change in clinical status of the patient, and/or (c) new clinical findings on cardiac examination [28].

Inappropriate reasons for performing TTE include transient fever (without bacteremia or new murmur) and cases of transient bacteremia with a non-IE pathogen and/or documentation of noncardiovascular infection. Also, performing echocardiography for routine surveillance without complications or when findings would not change management, is considered inappropriate and should be avoided [28].

3.1.2. Transesophageal imaging

Appropriateness guidelines for the use of TEE are more generic and are not necessarily specific for endocarditis. The use of TEE is considered reasonable in the following situations: (a) it is anticipated TTE imaging would be suboptimal, (b) to assess for interval change, if it is likely to guide a change in therapy, (c) assess valvular structure for planned interventions, and (d) to diagnose endocarditis if moderate pretest probability in certain subgroups, such as staphylococcal bacteremia or fungemia, prosthetic valves or intracardiac devices [28].

Inappropriate indications include the following: (a) if TTE is likely to be diagnostic, (b) follow-up TEE, when anticipated it would not change therapy, and (c) to diagnose IE with a low pretest probability [28].

3.2. European-based guidelines

The 2015 European Society of Cardiology (ESC) Guidelines on the management of IE provide an alternative set of guidelines on the appropriate use of echocardiography, grouped according to management stage of the illness [17]. A summary of the guideline is provided as follows:

3.2.1. Diagnosis

Class I indications include the following: (a) TTE first line in suspected IE, (b) TEE if negative TTE or nondiagnostic but clinical suspicion of IE, (c) TEE if clinical suspicion of IE if prosthetic valve or cardiac device is present, (d) repeat TTE and/or TEE if initial examination negative but high-clinical suspicion.

Class IIa indications include the following: (a) consider echo for *Staphylococcus aureus* bacteremia and (b) consider TEE in all suspected cases of IE regardless of TTE findings, unless high-quality study of native right-sided uncomplicated infection.

3.2.2. Follow-up during medical therapy

A class I indication to repeat either TTE and/or TEE is recommended if a new complication is clinically suspected. Consideration to repeat the TTE and/or TEE without complication is given a class IIa indication. The reasoning relates to the possibility of detecting a clinically silent complication and the ability to monitor vegetation size. This class IIa recommendation suggests the frequency of serial imaging should be based on factors such as the initial pathology, type of organism, and the response to treatment.

3.2.3. Intraoperative echocardiography and follow-up after completion of therapy

Class I indications include the following: (a) Each patient should undergo intraoperative echocardiography and (b) follow-up TTE should be performed at the completion of antibiotic therapy.

It is also recommended TTE be performed on a periodic basis along with clinical assessment during the first 12 months following discharge to monitor for the development of heart failure [17]. Consideration should be given to repeat TTE at 1, 3, 6, and 12 months [1].

3.3. Summary of guidelines

The American and European guidelines are similar in most regards; however, the ESC recommendations place emphasis on performing TTE on all patients with suspected IE and suggest consideration be given to progress imaging during the course of treatment, even when there is no change in clinical status. These guidelines are important to provide physicians with direction on the appropriateness of imaging referrals.

4. Important subgroups of endocarditis

4.1. Prosthetic valve endocarditis

Prosthetic valve endocarditis incidence is estimated at 0.3–1.2% per patient-year and accounts for approximately 10–30% of all cases of IE [6, 29]. Infection is classified as early or late PVE (>12 months postsurgery) and is associated with a different microbiological profile [30]. The infection rates are similar for mechanical and bioprosthetic valves, although lower for mitral valve repair [6, 31, 32]. A large multicenter registry study found that the incidence of endocarditis in transcatheter aortic valve implantation (TAVI) was 0.5% by 12 months, with almost half of the patients not surviving to discharge [33].

Mechanical prostheses are prone to periannular complications due to infection of the sewing ring predisposing to abscess, fistula, and/or dehiscence and are more likely to occur within the first few months postsurgery. Bioprosthetic valves primarily seed vegetations on the leaflets which may progress to ulceration, perforation, and/or leaflet destruction [34].

Echocardiographic imaging is more challenging in PVE, particularly with mechanical valves, due to reverberation and acoustic shadowing. Periannular involvement is common and may be obscured by artifact from the valve prosthesis [34]. Mechanical prosthetic valves are susceptible to formation of adherent thrombus and pannus, while bioprosthetic valves degenerate over time and can develop tissue strands or leaflet tears which can mimic vegetations [35].

Transesophageal echo is superior for assessment and detection of mitral and aortic prosthetic valve abnormalities, including endocarditis, thrombus, and degenerative changes, particularly for mechanical prosthetic valves [36]. Imaging with TTE is limited by the availability of an acoustic window, intervening anatomical structures between the probe and the heart, lower transducer frequency, and acoustic shadowing [36]. Multiplane TEE is highly effective for detecting mechanical valve periprosthetic mitral regurgitation (**Figure 9**), unlike TTE in which acoustic artifact obscures the left atrial aspect of the image [37].

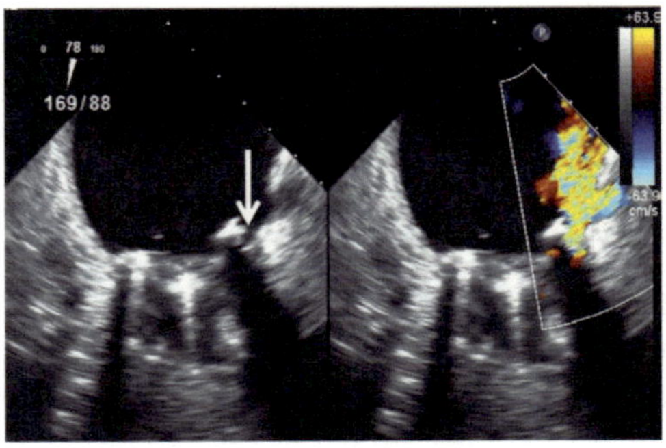

Figure 9. TEE color compare showing prosthetic annular dehiscence (arrow) associated with significant mitral regurgitation.

Although color and spectral Doppler assessment of prosthetic valves should be performed during TTE and TEE examinations, transthoracic echo is preferred for assessment of hemodynamics. In the case of a mechanical prosthetic aortic valve, TTE is also superior when assessing the anterior aortic root for abscess as acoustic shadowing is posteriorly directed obscuring the TEE image.

Aortic and mitral mechanical valve occluder motion is difficult to assess with TTE. The use of 2D and 3D TEE offers excellent assessment of mitral occluder motion; however, it is often suboptimal at visualizing the aortic occluders. The addition of cine fluoroscopy can definitively assess occluder-opening angles, while multidetector-row computed tomography (MDCT) is useful for evaluating occluder motion and identifying any mass lesions [38].

4.2. Right-sided endocarditis

Right-sided endocarditis (RSE) is epidemiologically distinct from left-sided cardiac infection and is associated with a lower mortality, except when vegetations are ≥20 mm [39]. Often vegetations are larger in size nevertheless infrequently associated with periannular extension [40].

The three major subgroups of RSE include IVDAs, cardiac device-related IE (CDRIE), and CHD. A minority of cases do not fit into any category, usually occurring in patients with structurally normal valves and a history of an indwelling venous catheter for treatment of an unrelated medical condition. This group may have a higher risk of periannular complications. In addition, left-sided IE, such as periannular aortic infection, can extend to involve the right-sided cardiac valves [40].

Endocarditis in IVDAs is more frequently associated with fungal and polymicrobial infections, both of which carry a much higher mortality than the expected 5–10% in RSE [39]. Endocarditis in the IVDA group most commonly involves the tricuspid valve with *S. aureus* the usual culprit. Infection rates are higher in HIV-seropositive and HIV-immunosuppressed individuals [40].

4.3. Cardiac device-related infections

Cardiac device-related endocarditis occurs in patients with pacemakers or implantable cardiac defibrillators, which are more prevalent in the older patient cohort. Endocarditis usually involves the presence of vegetations on the device lead, valves, or mural endocardium. Infective endocarditis must be distinguished from localized pocket site infection.

Echocardiography is fundamental for early diagnosis of CDRIE; nonetheless, it can be technically challenging due to artifact shadowing from the pacing leads. Transesophageal imaging is usually required and permits visualization of the leads, venae cavae, and high right atrial wall, which are often difficult to comprehensively investigate with TTE.

Small strands known as accretions are noted incidentally on device leads in approximately 30% of patients without clinical evidence of IE [41, 42]. The lesions appear as thin (1–2 mm) strands or occasionally as fixed small nodular echogenic structures on the leads and are not associated with a poorer prognosis [41].

4.4. Congenital heart disease

The incidence of IE in children is estimated at 0.34–0.64 per 100,000 person years, respectively, approximately ten times less common than in adults. Underlying CHD is found in 11–13% of adults with IE [43]. The most common underlying risk factor in children for endocarditis is CHD, followed by indwelling catheters. Rheumatic heart disease is now rare in developed countries. Only 2–5% of cases of IE occur in children with structurally normal valves compared to 25–45% of adults [44].

The main advantage of TTE over TEE is the need for anesthesia and intubation is avoided [44]. Transesophageal echocardiography should be utilized when TTE is negative but a high-clinical suspicion of IE remains, especially for periannular complications [45]. There are limited data comparing TEE with TTE in adult CHD. Both TTE and TEE may not adequately visualize vegetations or periannular complications associated with prosthetic shunts and conduits. Cardiac CT or MRI could be helpful in this setting [46].

5. Diagnostic accuracy

5.1. M-mode echocardiography

The first moving pictures of the heart using an ultrasound reflectoscope were recorded and published in 1953, by the 'father of echocardiography' Inge Edler, along with physicist Hellmuth Hertz. This led to the development of the standard time–motion (M-mode) ultrasonoscope, which later became known as an echocardiogram and depicted a single-imaging dimension displayed along a time axis [47].

Reference	No. of patients	No. of Vg or valves involved by gold standard*	Sensitivity and specificity for Vg	TTE NV (%)	PV (%)	PV (%) NV +	TEE NV (%)	PV (%)	NV + PV (%)	
Stafford et al. [53]	$n = 62$	$n = 29$ Sx/path	sens		–	–	93	–	–	–
			spec		–	–	89	–	–	–
Erbel et al. [54]	$n = 96$	AV = 15 MV = 3 PPM = 1 Sx/path	sens		63	–	–	100	–	–
			spec		98	–	–	98	–	–
Mügge et al. [55]	$n = 105$	NV = 69 PV = 22 Sx/path	sens	D	68	27	58	94	77	90
				P	90	36	77	100	86	97
			spec		–	–	–	–	–	–
Daniel et al. [36]	$n = 126$	PV = 33 Sx/path	sens		–	36	–	–	82	–
			spec		–	–	–	–	–	–
Shapiro et al. [56]	$n = 64$	NV+ PV = 30 TTE + TEE	sens		–	–	60	–	–	87
			spec		–	–	–	–	–	–
Lowry et al. [57]	$n = 93$	Clinical ± path ($n = 29$)	sens		50	17	36	100*	83*	93*
			spec		78	94	83	89*	95*	91*
Irani et al. [58]	$n = 134$	$n = 60$# TEE*	sens		68	–	–	–	–	–
			spec		100	–	–	–	–	–

Vg's = vegetations; TTE = transthoracic echocardiography; TEE = transesophageal echocardiography; NV = native valve; PV = prosthetic valve; n = number; Sx = surgery; path = pathological diagnosis, either surgical tissue or at autopsy; AV = aortic valve; MV= mitral valve; PPM = pacemaker lead; sens = sensitivity; spec = specificity; D = definite vegetations seen on echocardiography; P = possible vegetations in addition to definite vegetations seen on echocardiography. *Includes studies using biplane and/or multiplane TEE; # total number included vegetations and/or abscesses detected by TEE

Table 1. Diagnostic accuracy of TTE and TEE for detection of predominantly left-sided cardiac vegetations, pre harmonic era TTE imaging.

The first study to demonstrate vegetations using M-mode echocardiography was published in 1973 [48], followed by a case report of a tricuspid valve vegetation detected in 1974 [49]. Early work demonstrated M-mode was able to detect approximately one-third of native valve vegetations in patients with a clinical and/or pathological diagnosis of IE [50, 51].

Real-time 2D and 3D echocardiographic imaging, along with color and spectral Doppler capabilities, has superseded M-mode. The culmination of these advancements has enabled echocardiography to emerge as the imaging gold standard for IE and as such, be incorporated into the modified Duke [2] as a major diagnostic criterion. M-mode now contributes little to imaging in IE, except to demonstrate the typical vibrations of vegetations and/or prolapse of valvular tissue with high-temporal resolution (>1000 Hz cf. 30–60 Hz with 2D).

Reference	Gold standard*	Valve type	TEE—number of involved valves or vegetations by location					Sens TTE %	Spec TTE %
			NV	PV	PPM lead	Other site	Total		
Barton et al. [61]	TEE	NV + PV	MV = 50 AV = 34 TV = 19	MV = 16 AV = 25	*n* = 11	n = 1	n = 156	58 68#	–
Kini et al. [62]	TEE	NV + PV	n/a	*n* = 51	n/a	n/a	*n* = 179	45	79
Casella et al. [63]	TEE	NV	AV = 21 MV = 15 TV = 2					87 82^	86 62^
Jassal et al. [64]	TEE	NV	AV = 13 MV = 6	–	–	–	*n* = 19	84	88
Chirillo et al. [65]	TEE	NV + PV	AV = 11 MV = 10 TV = 3	AV = 3 MV = 6	–	–	*n* = 33	82 (HI) 36 (FI)	98 (HI) 80 (FI)
Reynolds et al, [66]	TEE	NV	AV=24 MV=26 TV=1	–	*n* = 2	*n* = 2	n=55 (valves, n= 51)	55	–

Vg's = vegetations; TTE = transthoracic echocardiography; TEE = transesophageal echocardiography; NV = native valve; PV = prosthetic valve; n = number; AV = aortic valve; MV= mitral valve; TV = tricuspid valve; n/a = not available; sens = sensitivity; spec = specificity; HI = harmonic imaging; FI = fundamental imaging. *modality against which sensitivity of TTE was compared; ^Included both definite and intermediate likelihood of IE on echocardiography; # sensitivity of TTE for detection of native valve vegetations, excluding prosthetic intracardiac material.

Table 2. Diagnostic accuracy of TTE compared to TEE for detection of predominantly left-sided cardiac vegetations utilizing modern era tissue harmonic imaging.

5.2. Transthoracic echocardiography

In the early 1970s real-time, phased array 2D TTE transducer technology was introduced, providing spatial resolution and anatomical detail not previously seen. This provided not only the ability to identify vegetations like its predecessor M-mode, but to accurately describe the size, point of attachment and morphology of intracardiac masses [52].

5.2.1. Vegetations

During the 1980s and 1990s, numerous landmark studies were published comparing the diagnostic accuracy of TTE for identification of predominantly left-sided cardiac vegetations.

Transthoracic echo was shown to have a combined sensitivity of 36–93% for native and prosthetic valve vegetations and a specificity of 78–100% (**Table 1**).

5.2.1.1. Harmonic tissue imaging

Harmonic sound waves are reflected back to the transducer at twice the frequency of the transmitted wave (fundamental frequency) and are subject to less near-field distortion and side lobe artifact. This results in a better signal-to-noise ratio with superior image resolution [47]. Specifically, there is an improvement in endocardial definition and visualization of the cardiac valves. However, the valve leaflet tissue itself may appear abnormally thickened when viewed using harmonic imaging [59, 60].

A number of studies have revisited the question of diagnostic accuracy of TTE for identification of mostly left-sided native valvular vegetations by comparing findings directly with TEE using modern era tissue harmonic imaging (hTTE). It remains unclear if modern era TTE imaging has resulted in improved detection of vegetations for left-sided vegetations, due to the wide variation in results reported (**Table 2**).

Reference	Gold standard*	No. abscesses confirmed by gold standard*	TEE multi-plane#	Sensitivity & Specificity	TTE			TEE		
					NV	PV	NV +PV	NV	PV	NV + PV
Daniel et al. [67]	Sx	46 (NV + PV)	No	sens	–	–	28	–	–	87
				spec	–	–	99	–	–	95
Aguado et al. [15]	Sx/path	25 (NV) 11 (PV)	No	sens	–	64	81	–	–	–
				spec	–	–	85	–	–	–
Choussat et al. [12]	Sx	64 (NV) 43 (PV)	Yes	sens	33	40	36	75	88	80
				spec	–	–	–	–	–	–
San Román et al. [24]	Sx/path	30 (PV)	Yes	sens	–	–	–	–	90	–
				spec	–	–	–	–	100	–
Cicioni et al. [68]	Sx	29 (NV + PV)	Yes	sens	–	–	38	–	–	93
				spec	–	–	–	–	–	–

TTE = transthoracic echocardiography; TEE = transesophageal echocardiography; NV = native valve; PV = prosthetic valve; sens = sensitivity; spec = specificity; Sx = surgery; path = pathology, either confirmed with surgery or at autopsy. *modality against which sensitivity and specificity of TTE and/or TEE was compared against. #Multiplane TEE probe transducer utilised for imaging in some or all patients in a study.

Table 3. Diagnostic accuracy of TTE and TEE for detection of abscess.

5.2.2. Abscess

Published data on diagnostic accuracy vary widely for abscess detection by TTE. Sensitivity has been reported at 28–81% with specificity 85–100% (**Table 3**). It is uncertain if harmonic imaging has positively impacted on the diagnostic accuracy, with some studies reporting no improvement [65, 68].

5.2.3. Other complications

There are limited studies, generally with small patient cohorts, assessing the diagnostic accuracy of echocardiography for identifying complications other than vegetation and abscess.

Information regarding accuracy of TTE for identifying pseudoaneurysms is sparse, mostly because this pathological finding is often included in with the abscess group. According to one publication, only about one-half of intervalvular pseudoaneurysms were correctly diagnosed by TTE [21].

The sensitivity of TTE is approximately 50% [23] for detection of aorto-cavitary fistulas, but as high as 93% for detecting periannular dehiscence [68]. Detection rates for perforations with TTE range from 45 to 75% [68, 70, 71] and similar for valve aneurysms (38–75%) when compared with TEE as the gold standard [20, 72]. Not surprisingly valve aneurysms are most likely to be missed on TTE when small in size [21, 73].

Reference	Cohort	Number of patients	Gold standard *	Diagnostic sensitivity of imaging modality			
				M-Mode %	2D TTE %	2D TEE %	ICE %
Berger et al. [75]	IVDA	12	Clinical	60	83	–	–
Ginzton et al. [76]	IVDA#	16	Clinical	63	100		–
Klug et al. [77]	CDRIE	52	Clinical ± Sx	–	23	94	–
Cacoub et al. [78]	CDRIE	33	Clinical ± Sx	–	22	96	–
Victor et al. [42]	CDRIE	23	Clinical ± micro	–	30	91	–
Narducci et al. [79]	CDRIE	44	Clinical ('definite'IE group)	–	–	73	100

IVDA = intravenous drug abuse; CDRIE = cardiac device-related infective endocarditis; TTE = transthoracic echocardiography; TEE = transesophageal echocardiography; ICE = intracardiac echocardiography; sens = sensitivity; spec = specificity; Sx = surgery; micro = microbiological diagnosis. *modality against which sensitivity and specificity of echocardiography was compared against; #majority of patient cohort were IVDA

Table 4. Diagnostic accuracy of TTE and TEE for right-sided valvular and cardiac device-related vegetations.

5.2.4. Subgroups of endocarditis

Limited data have been published addressing the sensitivity of TTE in RSE [74]. For tricuspid valve IE, mostly in the IVDA cohort, sensitivity is high at 83–100% [75, 76], while detection rates in CDRIE are poor at 22–30% (**Table 4**). Transthoracic echo may be adequate for isolated native tricuspid valve IE, especially in IVDAs, unless image quality is suboptimal or if clinical suspicion remains despite negative TTE. Transesophageal echo should be utilized if there may be periannular infection, pulmonary, or left-sided valvular involvement or in the presence of an indwelling intravenous catheter [40].

The sensitivity of echocardiography for diagnosis of IE in CHD overall is estimated at 60–80%, but less sensitive if complex pathology is present [46]. In one study, approximately one-third of adult patients with CHD and a clinical diagnosis of IE had negative findings on TTE and/or TEE and up to 70% of echocardiograms were negative in palliated complex conditions [80].

In young children, TTE is often sufficient to diagnose IE due to superior acoustic windows compared to adults. Transthoracic echo in children with IE has a high rate of detection of vegetations (>90%) when compared with TEE as the gold standard [81].

5.3. Transesophageal echocardiography

Transesophageal echo using monoplane imaging transducers was introduced into clinical practice in the early 1980s. The spatial resolution and utility of 2D TEE has continued to improve with the introduction of biplane and subsequent multiplane TEE transducers along with other advances in probe technology, digital processing, and image display.

5.3.1. Vegetations

During the 1980s and 1990s, with the introduction of monoplane TEE, a number of landmark studies were published comparing the diagnostic accuracy of TEE for identification of vegetations against the gold standard of surgery or pathological findings. Reported sensitivities and specificities of TEE for detection of left-sided vegetations ranged from 94 to 100% and 77 to 95% for native and prosthetic valves, respectively. Specificity was consistently high at >90% (**Table 1**).

A few studies compared monoplane, biplane, and multiplane TEE. Earlier work found marginally higher detection rates of vegetations and/or abscesses, but differences were minimal [82, 83]. Monoplane TEE not only underestimated vegetation size and extent but also was found to be less accurate at detecting small vegetations [83]. Contemporary studies using multiplane imaging report sensitivities >90% [68, 84]. Considering TEE imaging has always demonstrated high sensitivity and specificity for detection of vegetations, it is unclear if multiplane imaging has improved the diagnostic accuracy.

The reported sensitivity of 2D TEE for detection of vegetations in CDRIE ranges from 73 to 96% (**Table 4**) and is also superior over TTE for distinguishing site of attachment, whether valvular or on a lead.

5.3.2. Abscess

Three landmark studies from the 1990s investigated diagnosis of abscess by echocardiography comparing findings with surgery or autopsy. Daniel et al. [67], Choussat et al. [12], and San Román et al. [24] found that the sensitivity of TEE for abscess was 87, 80, and 90%, respectively. However, other studies have reported greater variability, with sensitivities ranging from 48 to 93%. Specificity has consistently remained high at >90% (**Table 3**).

It is unclear whether detection rates for abscesses have improved since the introduction of multiplane TEE. Although more recent studies in **Table 3** utilized biplane and multiplane imaging, the results did not demonstrate a significant improvement in diagnostic accuracy.

5.3.3. Other complications

Similar to TTE, there are limited studies with small patient cohorts assessing the diagnostic accuracy of TEE for identifying the complications of IE, other than vegetation and abscess.

Accurate detection of perforations is relatively high, ranging from 75 to 100% [68, 70, 71]. Transesophageal echo is the imaging modality of choice for identifying valve aneurysms, although sensitivity is unknown [73, 85], while aorto-cavitary fistulas are almost always identified correctly, with a sensitivity of 97–100% [23, 24]. Perivalvular dehiscence can be accurately diagnosed in the majority of cases with a sensitivity of 71–100% [68, 69, 86, 87] and specificity of >90% [69].

5.4. Three-dimensional echocardiography

Three-dimensional TTE and TEE have been part of clinical practice now in excess of 10 years. Over time, equipment has dramatically improved with the latest TEE matrix array transducers composed of up to almost 3000 piezoelectric elements. This leap of technology has been accompanied by improved digital processing power and miniaturization, along with other software and hardware improvements.

Three-dimensional echocardiography provides a choice of acquisition modes including multiplane (X-plane), real-time 'live' 3D, full-volume (stitched or single beat) 3D, zoom 3D and 3D color Doppler. Live 3D and 3D zoom modes are single-beat acquisitions and represent cardiac structure and function in real time. Full-volume acquisitions have the option of 'stitching' sequential volume datasets over a few cardiac cycles, providing a larger field of view. Single-beat full volume is available; however, it is limited by reduced temporal and spatial resolution.

5.4.1. Vegetation

The role of 3D echocardiographic imaging of vegetations is not well studied. A few case reports or small series confirm, as would be expected, that 3D TEE provides better morphological characterization and localization of lesions compared to 2D TEE. Three-dimensional TEE was shown to improve detection of vegetations in some case reports [88–91]; however, small vegetations may theoretically be more reliably detected with 2D due to higher temporal and spatial resolution.

A major benefit of 3D is the ability to visualize the entire valve and annulus in a single beat, enabling identification of eccentrically located vegetations that may otherwise be missed on a standard 2D TEE examination. Also, 3D imaging provides more accurate assessment of vegetation size. In a direct comparison by Berdejo et al. [92], mitral vegetation length of ≥16 mm on 2D and ≥20 mm with 3D best predicted embolic events.

5.4.2. Abscess

There are no published data to reliably estimate the diagnostic accuracy of 3D TTE or TEE for detection of abscess. However, 3D TEE imaging has been shown in case reports to provide useful additional information regarding the periannular extent of abscess and the relation to surrounding anatomical structures, including the coronary arteries [90, 93].

5.4.3. Other complications

Three-dimensional imaging enables valve perforations to be viewed 'en face' providing precise localization and sizing of any defect, while a small number of case reports indicate a higher detection rate when compared to 2D TEE [94, 95]. One drawback of 3D is artifactual 'dropout', especially with thin valvular tissue and suboptimal gain settings, which can result in false-positive findings. To confirm the finding, the defect should be visualized in systole and diastole and associated with a thickened rim surrounding the perforation [96]. Finally, 3D may assist with surgical planning when repair is contemplated [94, 96].

Three-dimensional TEE has the potential to demonstrate the extent and location of a valve aneurysm with greater accuracy than 2D imaging [97]. Similarly with perivalvular dehiscence, 3D is able to define the anatomic spatial relationship to surrounding structures and accurately define the location, size, and extent of the pathology [93]. One study showed the added benefit of 3D contrast TTE for accurately delineating the size and extent of a left ventricular pseudoaneurysm, when compared to 2D contrast TTE [98].

The role of 3D echo for right-sided IE is restricted to case reports and small case series [99, 100]. Sungur et al. [101] published the first study that compared 3D versus 2D TEE in tricuspid valve endocarditis against the gold standard of surgery. Three-dimensional imaging provided en-face visualization of all three TV leaflets in nine of 10 cases, allowing accurate identification and localization of multiple vegetations. In addition, 3D was able to better characterize vegetation morphology and size. Three-dimensional TEE also identified a tricuspid annular abscess that was missed on 2D TEE imaging. Three-dimensional TEE may add incremental value in localizing vegetations that are partly obscured by reverberation artifact on 2D imaging [99]. Because the right heart is located anteriorly in the chest, 3D TTE is particularly useful and has the potential to provide better imaging of the tricuspid valve.

5.5. Limitations of echocardiography

Echocardiography, especially TTE, has a number of potential limitations due to patient and nonpatient factors. TTE image quality is influenced by body habitus, chest wall deformity, rib space size, and interposing lung tissue. Poor TTE image quality is the main factor accounting for the superior diagnostic accuracy of TEE [54].

Furthermore, the skills of the sonographer and echocardiologist also influence diagnostic accuracy as shown by interobserver variability. Clinical history is important to the reporting echocardiographer but may result in bias with a trade-off between sensitivity and specificity [102, 103].

The ultrasound equipment, machine settings, and transducer frequency all impact on diagnostic accuracy. The limits of image resolution allow detection of vegetations down to 1.5–2 and 3–4 mm, for TEE and TTE, respectively. Not surprisingly, it has been shown that smaller vegetation size reduces the sensitivity of TTE [54, 104].

Mimickers of vegetations are often responsible for false-positive findings. Examples include degenerative valvular tissue, calcification, flail chords, thrombus, tumor, artifact from calcium or prosthetic material, and even normal anatomical variants such as a prominent Eustachian valve. Small thin linear strands are common and are frequently seen on native valves along the leaflet coaptation zone and may be confused with vegetations. Also, small sterile strands are frequently (18–43%) seen on prosthetic valves and are of uncertain significance [105].

The limitations outlined underscore the need to repeat imaging in due course (usually within one week) if the initial TTE and TEE are both negative, but there remains ongoing clinical suspicion of IE.

6. Echocardiographic predictors of prognosis

Embolism occurs in approximately one-quarter to one-half of patients [106, 107] with endocarditis, but the risk is substantially reduced after initiation of antibiotics within the first 1–2 weeks [111, 114]. Large mobile vegetations are associated with more complications. Vegetations >10 mm in length [55, 106, 110] and mobile masses carry the greatest risks of embolism [106, 111, 112].

Vegetations >15 mm and high mobility pose a major risk of systemic embolism [113]. Previous embolism, change in size of vegetations, *S. aureus*, and mitral valve location increase the risk of new embolism [114]. Right-sided vegetations ≥20 mm portend a poor prognosis, with mortality similar to that of left-sided IE [39, 40].

Echocardiography is very useful at identifying important prognostic markers related to extent of infection, cardiac function, and hemodynamics. Predictors of outcome include periannular extension, severe valvular dysfunction, left and right ventricular systolic function, left atrial size, left ventricular size, left ventricular filling pressures, and pulmonary artery pressure [1, 110, 115, 116]. More specifically, in left-sided native valve *S. aureus* endocarditis, an LVEF <40% or presence of abscess independently predicts in-hospital mortality while abscess and leaflet perforation both independently predict 12-month mortality [117].

7. Surgery and the role of echocardiography

Although patients may respond to prolonged antibiotic therapy alone, up to 50% will require surgical intervention [118]. Early surgery within the first week of antimicrobial therapy can improve survival in complicated left-sided IE; however, it may increase the risk of relapse and prosthetic valve dysfunction [119]. Echocardiography is fundamental in identifying important complications and prognostic markers that influence the timing of surgery.

Heart failure and embolism are the leading causes of mortality. Early surgery for left-sided IE is generally indicated in the following circumstances: (a) congestive cardiac failure, (b) periannular extension, for example, abscess and fistula, (c) large vegetations (>30 mm or possibly >15 mm) or recurrent emboli (>10 mm), (d) difficult to treat organisms such as *S. aureus*, multiresistant microbes, or fungi, (e) prosthetic valve endocarditis especially with Gram-negative, non-HACEK organisms, and (f) persistent sepsis or uncontrolled intracardiac infection including enlarging vegetations, despite appropriate antibiotics [17, 27].

Perioperative pre-pump 2D and 3D TEE provides the surgeon with a comprehensive real-time assessment of the extent of intracardiac pathology and cardiac hemodynamic status immediately prior to the procedure. A decision can be made on the feasibility of repair versus valve replacement and allows planning of the surgical strategy. The postpump TEE assesses cardiac function, hemodynamics, and the adequacy of surgical procedure. In addition, imaging can ensure the heart is appropriately 'de-aired' prior to removal of the cardiac vent. Intraoperative TEE for IE has been shown to positively impact on at least one of these factors in approximately one-third of operations [120].

8. Image optimization

8.1. Two-dimensional echocardiography

Image optimization is particularly important in IE to ensure early diagnosis and accurate identification of complications. Despite advances in TTE imaging quality, TEE still provides superior diagnostic capability. A TEE probe is in close proximity to the heart, with minimal intervening tissues and therefore less attenuation of the ultrasound waves. This allows the use of a higher frequency (5–7.5 MHz) transducer and provides superior spatial resolution.

The same principles of image optimization apply to both TTE and TEE. To obtain superior spatial resolution, select the highest frequency transducer that will maintain adequate depth penetration. Position the focal zone adjacent to the region of interest and adjust depth and sector width to optimize spatial and temporal resolution [47, 121]. Gain, time gain compensation (TGC), and dynamic compression of the gray scale are adjusted to optimize image contrast, while zoom function in real time improves spatial and temporal resolution [122].

8.2. Three-dimensional echocardiography

Three-dimensional image resolution is dependent on the quality of the 2D picture; therefore, optimizing the image prior to changing to 3D mode is essential. Select the imaging plane or acoustic window with the highest resolution. Imaging in the axial plane provides superior resolution (0.5–1 mm) followed by lateral (1.5–2 mm) and finally elevational resolution (2.5–3 mm) [123]. When performing 3D TTE, select the window that transects the structure of interest through the axial and lateral plane such as the parasternal long axis for the mitral valve.

To allow for optimal postprocessing, it is recommended the gain, compensation, and compression be in the midrange, with the TGC adjusted to display a uniform, slightly brighter image [124]. As spatial resolution increases, temporal resolution is reduced and vice versa. This is due to the limited number of scan lines that can be performed in a fixed period of time.

http://dx.doi.org/10.5772/64800

To improve image resolution, narrow the sector width and optimize frequency, compression, and focus [124, 125].

Multibeat 3D volume rendered image acquisition is limited by 'stitching' artifact from respiration and/or arrhythmia [124]. This can be addressed with breath holding and ensuring image acquisition during regular R-R intervals on the ECG.

Cropping of the 3D dataset can be performed en cart prior to image storage or alternatively, offline on a workstation using proprietary software. The 3D data can then be displayed as volume rendered format and surface rendered format or 2D tomographic slices [123].

Finally, the 3D rendered image is rotated and orientated according to convention. The mitral valve from the left atrial perspective (surgeon's view) with the aorta superiorly (12 o'clock), the aortic valve with the right coronary cusp inferiorly (6 o'clock), the tricuspid valve with the interventricular septum inferiorly (6 o'clock), and the pulmonary valve with the anterior cusp superiorly (12 o'clock). The display formats remain the same regardless of whether the valve is viewed from above or below [124].

9. Imaging protocol for infective endocarditis

Imaging for IE requires a methodical approach and follows the same principles for TTE and TEE. All standard TTE and/or TEE transducer positions and views should be obtained with meticulous scrutiny of the cardiac valves and periannular tissues. Use zoom mode to focus on each valve individually to ensure subtle pathology is not overlooked.

It is important to pan through the cardiac valves and adjacent supporting structures using multiple angles and off-axis imaging. This can be achieved with TEE probe manipulation, such as anteflexion, retroflexion, lateral flexion, probe turning, and probe advancement or withdrawal. Careful manipulation of the probe is required to avoid trauma or perforation of the upper gastrointestinal tract. Similarly, the TTE transducer can be angulated, rotated, or repositioned on the chest wall to maximize diagnostic utility.

With the introduction of multiplane TEE, the 2D image can be effortlessly rotated through 180 degrees. Thorough inspection of the valves, with 2D and color flow Doppler, should be undertaken at frequent intervals, as the angle is increased. This is particularly useful for detecting mitral annular complications and/or localized perivalvular regurgitation.

Interrogation of valvular function with color Doppler along with hemodynamic assessment is essential. Attention should be paid to abnormal color flow arising from valves, fistulae, or other shunts. Images along the direction and path of any pathological color flow are used to identify abnormal communications and exclude jet lesions. Assess cardiac chambers for mural vegetations and the vasculature for endarteritis.

Finally, it is imperative to complete a comprehensive echocardiographic study to assess cardiac function, hemodynamics, filling pressures, and pulmonary artery pressure.

Three-dimensional functionalities such as X-plane, real-time, and multibeat 3D should be routinely incorporated, especially for TEE examination of the mitral and aortic valves. Transthoracic 3D of the tricuspid valve is useful for assessing valve anatomy and pathology, particularly in patients with regurgitation associated with pacing leads [126]. For valvular complications of endocarditis, 3D zoom is preferred, providing good spatial and temporal resolution with a single-beat acquisition [123]. However, if assessing extensive perivalvular pathology or ventricular size and function, then change to a wide-angle full-volume 3D multibeat acquisition.

10. Quality control

Leading echocardiography laboratories must ensure that high standards are accomplished both for clinical practice and for scientific research. Recommendations for core laboratories, including quality control guidelines, have been published by the American Society of Echocardiography [108, 127] and European Association of Echocardiography (Cardiovascular Imaging) [128]. Periodic auditing of stored images and reports should be undertaken and reviewed by an experienced physician. Echocardiographic findings of endocarditis should undergo pathological correlation with surgery or a complimentary imaging modality, such as cardiac CT.

For a center to develop excellence in endocarditis management, a dedicated imaging and clinical database should be established for auditing, quality control, and research purposes. Recent guidelines recommend the establishment of a specialized multidisciplinary team at centers with expertise in managing IE [109]. This approach has been demonstrated to reduce mortality by over 50% [129]. The endocarditis team should be engaged early in the management of suspected IE and urgent echocardiography performed.

The lead echocardiologist should have expertise in the field of cardiac infection and provide ongoing education to medical colleagues and sonographers alike to ensure the highest imaging standards are met. When IE is suspected on echo, expert interpretation of the findings should be communicated urgently to the treating team, especially when significant pathology is identified. The echocardiologist is also able to advise of any requirement for a supplemental procedure, such as TEE or CT, and provide recommendations with regard to appropriate follow-up imaging [17, 27, 109, 130].

11. Complimentary imaging modalities and future directions

11.1. Intracardiac echocardiography

Intracardiac echocardiography (ICE) has the potential to provide better image quality than TEE due to its use of higher frequency ultrasound in close proximity to the right-sided cardiac structures. Narducci et al. [79] directly compared the two modalities, with ICE detecting more intracardiac masses than TEE (**Table 4**).

Consider using ICE, particularly in CDRIE where TEE is inconclusive or discordant with clinical findings. Although ICE is considered a safe procedure [131, 132], its routine use is limited by cost. Future applications include the use of 3D ICE and electroanatomic mapping [131].

11.2. Contrast echocardiography

The application of targeted microbubbles and molecular contrast imaging offers promise as an emerging field of research. Contrast agents could be designed to tag certain cellular or molecular markers, such as inflammatory cells or ligands, enabling contrast imaging to detect the presence, location, and extent of the targeted pathology [133].

11.3. Cardiac computed tomography

Multislice CT shows similar diagnostic performance to TEE for detection of large native and prosthetic valve vegetations, valve aneurysm, abscess, and pseudoaneurysm and provides superior anatomical detail relating to the extent of periannular extension and relation to surrounding structures. Vegetations ≤4 mm and small valvular leaflet perforations are not well detected by CT [84, 134–136]. CT is very helpful for imaging the coronary arteries prior to surgery and for detecting extracardiac complications of endocarditis [134]. A major drawback is the exposure to ionizing radiation.

11.4. Positron emission tomography and fusion imaging

There is interest also in nuclear molecular techniques, in particular ^{18}F-fluorodeoxyglucose (FDG) PET/CT or PET/CTA, as a complimentary modality to echocardiography, especially when TEE is negative in the very early stages of infection and clinical suspicion remains high [136, 137]. ^{18}F-FDG is taken up avidly by leukocytes and therefore identifies regions of inflammation. The CT scan provides complimentary anatomical information. The use of PET/CT has been shown to substantially improve the sensitivity and thus diagnostic utility of the modified Duke criteria for diagnosis of both prosthetic valve endocarditis and cardiac device-related infections [138].

11.5. Cardiac magnetic resonance imaging

Contrast cardiac MRI can potentially detect early periannular extension of infection and may also identify vegetations, although with less accuracy [139]. The role of cardiac MRI in this domain remains undefined. MRI is useful for diagnosing cerebral complications of IE [17, 136].

11.6. Molecular imaging

Potential techniques include bioluminescence and radiolabeled antibodies or leukocytes, to target bacteria, biofilms, fibrin, and sites of inflammation. Bioluminescence requires optical imaging, while radiolabeling uses PET, SPECT, or combined modalities [140]. These experimental techniques may have applications such as detection of infected vascular grafts or intracardiac infection [136].

12. Summary

Echocardiography is fundamental in the management of all aspects of endocarditis from diagnosis, identifying complications and prognostic factors through to guiding surgery, and providing follow-up after treatment. Over the past 40 years, since the introduction of M-mode, echocardiography has evolved rapidly, with high-quality 2D and 3D imaging now in routine clinical use. Echocardiography is readily available, cost-effective, and safe, without exposure to ionizing radiation.

Confirming the diagnosis of endocarditis has never been easier with modern era echo; however, mortality remains high, in part due to delayed diagnosis. Maintaining a high-clinical suspicion for IE in at-risk patients must be combined with early referral for echo to ensure prompt diagnosis and institution of appropriate therapy. Formation of an expert multidisciplinary IE team and appropriate use of echocardiography has the potential to save lives and improve patient outcomes.

Author details

John F. Sedgwick[1,2] and Gregory M. Scalia[1,2,3*]

*Address all correspondence to: gmscalia@gmail.com

1 Department of Echocardiography, Cardiology Program, The Prince Charles Hospital, Brisbane, QLD, Australia

2 The University of Queensland, Brisbane, Australia

3 Heart Care Partners, Brisbane, Australia

References

[1] Habib G, Badano L, Tribouilloy C, Vilacosta I, Zamorano JL, Galderisi M, et al. Recommendations for the practice of echocardiography in infective endocarditis. European Journal of Echocardiography: The Journal of the Working Group on Echocardiography of the European Society of Cardiology. 2010;11(2):202–19.

[2] Durack DT, Lukes AS, Bright DK. New criteria for diagnosis of infective endocarditis: utilization of specific echocardiographic findings. Duke Endocarditis Service. The American Journal of Medicine. 1994;96(3):200.

[3] Perez-Vazquez A, Farinas MC, Garcia-Palomo JD, Bernal JM, Revuelta JM, Gonzalez-Macias J. Evaluation of the duke criteria in 93 episodes of prosthetic valve endocarditis: could sensitivity be improved? Archives of Internal Medicine. 2000;160(8):1185–91.

[4] Sandre RM, Shafran SD. Infective endocarditis: review of 135 cases over 9 years. Clinical Infectious Diseases. 1996;22(2):276–86.

[5] Dodds GA, Sexton DJ, Durack DT, Bashore TM, Corey GR, Kisslo J, et al. Negative predictive value of the Duke criteria for infective endocarditis. The American Journal of Cardiology. 1996;77(5):403–7.

[6] Habib G, Hoen B, Tornos P, Thuny F, Prendergast B, Vilacosta I, et al. Guidelines on the prevention, diagnosis, and treatment of infective endocarditis (new version 2009). European Heart Journal. 2009;30(19):2369–413.

[7] Habib G, Derumeaux G, Avierinos J-F, Casalta J-P, Jamal F, Volot F, et al. Value and limitations of the duke criteria for the diagnosis of infective endocarditis. Journal of the American College of Cardiology. 1999;33(7):2023–9.

[8] Roe MT, Abramson MA, Li J, Heinle SK, Kisslo J, Corey GR, et al. Clinical information determines the impact of transesophageal echocardiography on the diagnosis of infective endocarditis by the duke criteria. American Heart Journal. 2000;139(6):945–51.

[9] Reisner SA, Brenner B, Haim N, Edoute Y, Markiewicz W. Echocardiography in nonbacterial thrombotic endocarditis: from autopsy to clinical entity. Journal of the American Society of Echocardiography: Official Publication of the American Society of Echocardiography. 2000;13(9):876.

[10] Liu J, Frishman W. Nonbacterial thrombotic endocarditis—pathogenesis, diagnosis and management. Cardiology in Review. 2016:1 244–247.

[11] Scalia GM, Tandon AK, Robertson JA. Stroke, aortic vegetations and disseminated adenocarcinoma—a case of marantic endocarditis. Heart, Lung and Circulation. 2012;21(4):234–6.

[12] Choussat R. Perivalvular abscesses associated with endocarditis clinical features and prognostic factors of overall survival in a series of 233 cases. European Heart Journal. 1999;20(3):232–41.

[13] Ellis SG, Goldstein J, Popp RL. Detection of endocarditis-associated perivalvular abscesses by two-dimensional echocardiography. Journal of the American College of Cardiology. 1985;5(3):647–53.

[14] Baumgartner FJ, Omari BO, Robertson JM, Nelson RJ, Pandya A, Pandya A, et al. Annular abscesses in surgical endocarditis: anatomic, clinical, and operative features. The Annals of Thoracic Surgery. 2000;70(2):442–7.

[15] Aguado JM, GonzÃ¡lez-VÃÂlchez F, MartÃÂn-DurÃ¡n R, Arjona R, Prada JAVzd. Perivalvular abscesses associated with endocarditis. Clinical features

and diagnostic accuracy of two-dimensional echocardiography. Chest. 1993;104(1): 88–93.

[16] Afridi I, Apostolidou MA, Saad RM, Zoghbi WA. Pseudoaneurysms of the mitral-aortic intervalvular fibrosa: dynamic characterization using transesophageal echocardiographic and Doppler techniques. Journal of the American College of Cardiology. 1995;25(1):137–45.

[17] Habib G, Lancellotti P, Antunes MJ, Bongiorni MG, Casalta J-P, Del Zotti F, et al. 2015 ESC guidelines for the management of infective endocarditis: The Task Force for the Management of Infective Endocarditis of the European Society of Cardiology (ESC)Endorsed by: European Association for Cardio-Thoracic Surgery (EACTS), the European Association of Nuclear Medicine (EANM). European Heart Journal. 2015;36(44):3075.

[18] Effron MK, Popp RL. Two-dimensional echocardiographic assessment of bioprosthetic valve dysfunction and infective endocarditis. Journal of the American College of Cardiology. 1983;2(4):597–606.

[19] Ballal RS, Mahan EF, Nanda NC, Sanyal R. Aortic and mitral valve perforation: diagnosis by transesophageal echocardiography and doppler color flow imaging. American Heart Journal. 1991;121(1):214–7.

[20] Vilacosta I, San Román JA, Sarriá C, Iturralde E, Graupner C, Batlle E, et al. Clinical, anatomic, and echocardiographic characteristics of aneurysms of the mitral valve. The American Journal of Cardiology. 1999;84(1):110–3.

[21] Karalis DG, Bansal RC, Hauck AJ, Ross JJJ, Applegate PM, Jutzy KR, et al. Transesophageal echocardiographic recognition of subaortic complications in aortic valve endocarditis. Clinical and surgical implications. Circulation. 1992;86(2):353–62.

[22] Anguera I, Quaglio G, Miró JM, Paré C, Azqueta M, Marco F, et al. Aortocardiac fistulas complicating infective endocarditis. The American Journal of Cardiology. 2001;87(5): 652–4.

[23] Anguera I, Miro JM, Vilacosta I, Almirante B, Anguita M, Muñoz P, et al. Aorto-cavitary fistulous tract formation in infective endocarditis: clinical and echocardiographic features of 76 cases and risk factors for mortality. European heart journal. 2005;26(3): 288–97.

[24] San Román JA, Vilacosta I, Sarriá C, de la Fuente L, Sanz O, Vega JL, et al. Clinical course, microbiologic profile, and diagnosis of periannular complications in prosthetic valve endocarditis. The American Journal of Cardiology. 1999;83(7):1075–9.

[25] O'Dowd CE, Garlick B, Bartley JP, Scalia GM. Perforated mitral valve annular phlegmon with ventriculo-atrial fistula. Heart, Lung & Circulation. 2013;22(3):221.

[26] Sudhakar S, Sewani A, Agrawal M, Uretsky BF. Pseudoaneurysm of the mitral-aortic intervalvular fibrosa (MAIVF): a comprehensive review. Journal of the American Society of Echocardiography. 2010;23(10):1009–18.

http://dx.doi.org/10.5772/64800

[27] Nishimura RA, Otto CM, Bonow RO, Carabello BA, Erwin JP, Guyton RA, et al. 2014 AHA/ACC guideline for the management of patients with valvular heart disease. Journal of the American College of Cardiology. 2014;63(22):e57–e185.

[28] Douglas PS, Garcia MJ, Haines DE, Lai WW, Manning WJ, Patel AR, et al. ACCF/ASE/AHA/ASNC/HFSA/HRS/SCAI/SCCM/SCCT/SCMR 2011 appropriate use criteria for echocardiography. Journal of the American College of Cardiology. 2011;57(9):1126–66.

[29] Wang A, Athan E, Pappas PA, Fowler JVG, Olaison L, Paré C, et al. Contemporary clinical profile and outcome of prosthetic valve endocarditis. JAMA. 2007;297(12):1354–61.

[30] López J, Revilla A, Vilacosta I, Villacorta E, González-Juanatey C, Gómez I, et al. Definition, clinical profile, microbiological spectrum, and prognostic factors of early-onset prosthetic valve endocarditis. European Heart Journal. 2007;28(6):760–5.

[31] Ruttmann E, Legit C, Poelzl G, Mueller S, Mueller LC, Chevtchik O, et al. Mitral valve repair provides improved outcome over replacement in active infective endocarditis. The Journal of Thoracic and Cardiovascular Surgery. 2005;130(3):765–71.

[32] Foster E. Mitral regurgitation due to degenerative mitral-valve disease. The New England Journal of Medicine. 2010;363(2):156–65.

[33] Amat-Santos IJ, Ribeiro HB, Urena M, Allende R, Houde C, Bédard E, et al. Prosthetic valve endocarditis after transcatheter valve replacement: a systematic review. JACC Cardiovascular Interventions 2015;8(2):334.

[34] Habib G, Thuny F, Avierinos J-F. Prosthetic valve endocarditis: current approach and therapeutic options. Progress in Cardiovascular Diseases. 2008;50(4):274–81.

[35] Tanabe K. Echocardiographic assessment of prosthetic valves. Journal of Echocardiography. 2015;13(4):126–33.

[36] Daniel WG, Mügge A, Grote J, Hausmann D, Nikutta P, Laas J, et al. Comparison of transthoracic and transesophageal echocardiography for detection of abnormalities of prosthetic and bioprosthetic valves in the mitral and aortic positions. The American Journal of Cardiology. 1993;71(2):210–5.

[37] Khandheria BK, Seward JB, Oh JK, Freeman WK, Nichols BA, Sinak LJ, et al. Value and limitations of transesophageal echocardiography in assessment of mitral valve prostheses. Circulation. 1991;83(6):1956–68.

[38] Tanis W, Budde RPJ, van der Bilt IAC, Delemarre B, Hoohenkerk G, van Rooden JK, et al. Novel imaging strategies for the detection of prosthetic heart valve obstruction and endocarditis. Netherlands Heart Journal. 2016;24(2):96–107.

[39] Martín-Dávila P, Navas E, Fortún J, Moya JL, Cobo J, Pintado V, et al. Analysis of mortality and risk factors associated with native valve endocarditis in drug users: the importance of vegetation size. American Heart Journal. 2005;150(5):1099–106.

[40] San Román JA, Vilacosta I, López J, Revilla A, Arnold R, Sevilla T, et al. Role of transthoracic and transesophageal echocardiography in right-sided endocarditis: one echocardiographic modality does not fit all. Journal of the American Society of Echocardiography: Official Publication of the American Society of Echocardiography. 2012;25(8):807.

[41] Dundar C, Tigen K, Tanalp C, Izgi A, Karaahmet T, Cevik C, et al. The prevalence of echocardiographic accretions on the leads of patients with permanent pacemakers. Journal of the American Society of Echocardiography. 2011;24(7):803–7.

[42] Victor F, De Place C, Camus C, Le Breton H, Leclercq C, Pavin D, et al. Pacemaker lead infection: echocardiographic features, management, and outcome. Heart (British Cardiac Society). 1999;81(1):82–7.

[43] Knirsch W, Nadal D. Infective endocarditis in congenital heart disease. European Journal of Pediatrics. 2011;170(9):1111–27.

[44] Wong PC, Miller-Hance WC, Silverman NH. Transesophageal Echocardiography for Congenital Heart Disease. London: Springer; 2014;399–436.

[45] Gómez-Núñez N, Vargas-Barrón J, Espinola-Zavaleta N, Romero-Cárdenas A, Hernández-Reyes P, Keirns C, et al. Echocardiographic study of patients with congenital heart disease and infective endocarditis. Echocardiography. 2001;18(6):485–90.

[46] Gatzoulis MA, Webb GD, Daubeney PEF. Diagnosis and Management of Adult Congenital Heart Disease. Philadelphia: Elsevier/Saunders; 2011;147–153.

[47] Edelman SK. Pulsed Echo Instrumentation. Understanding Ultrasound Physics, 4th ed. Woodlands, Tex: ESP; 2012. p. 215–38.

[48] Dillon JC, Feigenbaum H, Konecke LL, Davis RH, Chang S. Echocardiographic manifestations of valvular vegetations. American Heart Journal. 1973;86(5):698–704.

[49] Lee C-C, Ganguly SN, Magnisalis K, Robin E. Detection of tricuspid valve vegetations by echocardiography. Chest. 1974;66(4):432.

[50] Wann LS, Dillon JC, Weyman AE, Feigenbaum H. Echocardiography in bacterial endocarditis. The New England Journal of Medicine. 1976;295(3):135.

[51] Come PC, Isaacs RE, Riley MF. Diagnostic accuracy of M-mode echocardiography in active infective endocarditis and prognostic implications of ultrasound-detectable vegetations. American Heart Journal. 1982;103(5):839–47.

[52] Kisslo J. Comparison of M-mode and two-dimensional echocardiography. Circulation. 1979;60(4):734–6.

[53] Stafford WJ, Petch J, Radford DJ. Vegetations in infective endocarditis. Clinical relevance and diagnosis by cross sectional echocardiography. British heart journal. 1985;53(3):310–3.

[54] Erbel R, Rohmann S, Drexler M, Mohr-Kahaly S, Gerharz CD, Iversen S, et al. Improved diagnostic value of echocardiography in patients with infective endocarditis by transoesophageal approach. A prospective study. European Heart Journal. 1988;9(1): 43.

[55] Mügge A, Daniel WG, Frank G, Lichtlen PR. Echocardiography in infective endocarditis: reassessment of prognostic implications of vegetation size determined by the transthoracic and the transesophageal approach. Journal of the American College of Cardiology. 1989;14(3):631.

[56] Shapiro SM, Young E, Guzman SD, Ward J, Chiu CY, Ginzton LE, et al. Transesophageal echocardiography in diagnosis of infective endocarditis. Chest. 1994;105(2):377–82.

[57] Lowry RW, Zoghbi WA, Baker WB, Wray RA, Quinones MA. Clinical impact of transesophageal echocardiography in the diagnosis and management of infective endocarditis. American Journal of Cardiology. 1994;73(15):1089–91.

[58] Irani WN, Grayburn PA, Afridi I. A negative transthoracic echocardiogram obviates the need for transesophageal echocardiography in patients with suspected native valve active infective endocarditis. The American Journal of Cardiology. 1996;78(1): 101–3.

[59] Hawkins K, Henry JS, Krasuski RA. Original investigations: tissue harmonic imaging in echocardiography: better valve imaging, but at what cost?: tissue harmonics and valve imaging. Echocardiography. 2008;25(2):119–23.

[60] Caidahl K, Kazzam E, Lidberg J, Neumann-Andersen G, Nordanstig J, Dahlqvist SR, et al. New concept in echocardiography: harmonic imaging of tissue without use of contrast agent. The Lancet. 1998;352(9136):1264–70.

[61] Barton TL, Mottram PM, Stuart RL, Cameron JD, Moir S. Transthoracic echocardiography is still useful in the initial evaluation of patients with suspected infective endocarditis: evaluation of a large cohort at a tertiary referral center. Mayo Clinic Proceedings. 2014;89(6):799–805.

[62] Kini V. Transthoracic and transesophageal echocardiography for the indication of suspected infective endocarditis: vegetations, blood cultures and imaging. J Am Soc Echocardiogr. 2010;23(4):396–402.

[63] Casella F, Rana B, Casazza G, Bhan A, Kapetanakis S, Omigie J, et al. The potential impact of contemporary transthoracic echocardiography on the management of patients with native valve endocarditis: a comparison with transesophageal echocardiography. Echocardiography (Mount Kisco, NY). 2009;26(8):900.

[64] Jassal DS, Aminbakhsh A, Fang T, Shaikh N, Embil JM, Mackenzie GS, et al. Diagnostic value of harmonic transthoracic echocardiography in native valve infective endocarditis: comparison with transesophageal echocardiography. Cardiovascular Ultrasound. 2007;5(1):20.

[65] Chirillo F, Pedrocco A, De Leo A, Bruni A, Totis O, Meneghetti P, et al. Impact of harmonic imaging on transthoracic echocardiographic identification of infective endocarditis and its complications. Heart. 2005;91(3):329–33.

[66] Reynolds HR, Jagen MA, Tunick PA, Kronzon I. Sensitivity of transthoracic versus transesophageal echocardiography for the detection of native valve vegetations in the modern era. Journal of the American Society of Echocardiography. 2003;16(1):67–70.

[67] Daniel WG, Mügge A, Martin RP, Lindert O, Hausmann D, Nonnast-Daniel B, et al. Improvement in the diagnosis of abscesses associated with endocarditis by transesophageal echocardiography. The New England Journal of Medicine. 1991;324(12):795–800.

[68] Cicioni C, Di Luzio V, Di Emidio L, De Remigis F, Fragassi G, Gregorini R, et al. Limitations and discrepancies of transthoracic and transesophageal echocardiography compared with surgical findings in patients submitted to surgery for complications of infective endocarditis. Journal of Cardiovascular Medicine (Hagerstown, Md). 2006;7(9):660–6.

[69] Hill EE, Herijgers P, Claus P, Vanderschueren S, Peetermans WE, Herregods M-C. Abscess in infective endocarditis: the value of transesophageal echocardiography and outcome. American Heart Journal. 2007;154(5):923–8.

[70] De Castro S, Cartoni D, d'Amati G, Beni S, Yao J, Fiorell M, et al. Diagnostic accuracy of transthoracic and multiplane transesophageal echocardiography for valvular perforation in acute infective endocarditis: correlation with anatomic findings. Clinical Infectious Diseases. 2000;30(5):825–6.

[71] Cziner DG, Rosenzweig BP, Katz ES, Keller AM, Daniel WG, Kronzon I. Transesophageal versus transthoracic echocardiography for diagnosing mitral valve perforation. The American Journal of Cardiology. 1992;69(17):1495–7.

[72] Guler A, Karabay CY, Gursoy OM, Guler Y, Candan O, Akgun T, et al. Clinical and echocardiographic evaluation of mitral valve aneurysms: a retrospective, single center study. The International Journal of Cardiovascular Imaging. 2014;30(3):535–41.

[73] Mollod MDM, Felner KJ, Felner MDJM. Mitral and tricuspid valve aneurysms evaluated by transesophageal echocardiography. The American Journal of Cardiology. 1997;79(9):1269–72.

[74] Sedgwick JF, Burstow DJ. Update on echocardiography in the management of infective endocarditis. Current Infectious Disease Reports. 2012;14(4):373–80.

[75] Berger M, Delfin LA, Jelveh M, Goldberg E. Two-dimensional echocardiographic findings in right-sided infective endocarditis. Circulation. 1980;61(4):855–61.

[76] Ginzton LE, Siegel RJ, Criley JM. Natural history of tricuspid valve endocarditis: a two dimensional echocardiographic study. The American Journal of Cardiology. 1982;49(8):1853–9.

[77] Klug D, Lacroix D, Savoye C, Goullard L, Grandmougin D, Hennequin JL, et al. Systemic infection related to endocarditis on pacemaker leads: clinical presentation and management. Circulation. 1997;95(8):2098–107.

[78] Cacoub P, Leprince P, Nataf P, Hausfater P, Dorent R, Wechsler B, et al. Pacemaker infective endocarditis. The American Journal of Cardiology. 1998;82(4):480–4.

[79] Narducci ML, Pelargonio G, Russo E, Marinaccio L, Di Monaco A, Perna F, et al. Usefulness of intracardiac echocardiography for the diagnosis of cardiovascular implantable electronic device-related endocarditis. Journal of the American College of Cardiology. 2013;61(13):1398–405.

[80] Di Filippo S, Delahaye F, Semiond B, Celard M, Henaine R, Ninet J, et al. Current patterns of infective endocarditis in congenital heart disease. Heart (British Cardiac Society). 2006;92(10):1490–5.

[81] Humpl T, McCrindle BW, Smallhorn JF. The relative roles of transthoracic compared with transesophageal echocardiography in children with suspected infective endocarditis. Journal of the American College of Cardiology. 2003;41(11):2068–71.

[82] Tardif J-C, Schwartz SL, Vannan MA, Cao Q-L, Pandian NG. Clinical usefulness of multiplane transesophageal echocardiography: comparison to biplanar imaging. American Heart Journal. 1994;128(1):156–66.

[83] Job FP, Franke S, Lethen H, Flachskampf FA, Hanrath P. Incremental value of biplane and multiplane transesophageal echocardiography for the assessment of active infective endocarditis. The American Journal of Cardiology. 1995;75(15):1033–7.

[84] Feuchtner GM, Stolzmann P, Dichtl W, Schertler T, Bonatti J, Scheffel H, et al. Multislice computed tomography in infective endocarditis: comparison with transesophageal echocardiography and intraoperative findings. Journal of the American College of Cardiology. 2009;53(5):436.

[85] Karalis DG, Blumberg EA, Vilaro JF, Covalesky VA, Wahl JM, Chandrasekaran K, et al. Prognostic significance of valvular regurgitation in patients with infective endocarditis. The American Journal of Medicine. 1991;90(1):193–7.

[86] Fagman E, Perrotta S, Bech-Hanssen O, Flinck A, Lamm C, Olaison L, et al. ECG-gated computed tomography: a new role for patients with suspected aortic prosthetic valve endocarditis. European Radiology. 2012;22(11):2407–14.

[87] Habets J, Tanis W, Reitsma JB, van den Brink RBA, Mali WPTM, Chamuleau SAJ, et al. Are novel non-invasive imaging techniques needed in patients with suspected prosthetic heart valve endocarditis? A systematic review and meta-analysis. European Radiology. 2015;25(7):2125–33.

[88] Hansalia S, Biswas M, Dutta R, Hage FG, Hsiung MC, Nanda NC, et al. The value of live/real time three-dimensional transesophageal echocardiography in the assessment of valvular vegetations. Echocardiography. 2009;26(10):1264–73.

[89] de Isla LP, Zamorano J, Malangatana G, Almeria C, Rodrigo JL, Cordeiro P, et al. Usefulness of real-time 3-dimensional echocardiography in the assessment of infective endocarditis: initial experience. Journal of Ultrasound in Medicine. 2005;24(2):231.

[90] Tanis W, Teske AJ, Herwerden LA, Chamuleau S, Meijboom F, Budde RPJ, et al. The additional value of three-dimensional transesophageal echocardiography in complex aortic prosthetic heart valve endocarditis. Echocardiography. 2015;32(1):114–25.

[91] El Muayed M, Burjonroppa SC, Croitoru M. Added accuracy with 3D echocardiographic imaging of valvular vegetations. Echocardiography. 2005;22(4):361–2.

[92] Berdejo J, Shibayama K, Harada K, Tanaka J, Mihara H, Gurudevan SV, et al. Evaluation of vegetation size and its relationship with embolism in infective endocarditis: a real-time 3-dimensional transesophageal echocardiography study. Circulation: Cardiovascular Imaging. 2014;7(1):149–54.

[93] Mukhtari O, Horton CJ, Nanda NC, Aaluri SR, Pacifico A. Transesophageal color Doppler three-dimensional echocardiographic detection of prosthetic aortic valve dehiscence: correlation with surgical findings. Echocardiography. 2001;18(5):393–7.

[94] Bhave NM, Addetia K, Spencer KT, Weinert L, Jeevanandam V, Lang RM. Localizing mitral valve perforations with 3D transesophageal echocardiography. JACC Cardiovascular Imaging 2013;6(3):407.

[95] Thompson KA, Shiota T, Tolstrup K, Gurudevan SV, Siegel RJ. Utility of three-dimensional transesophageal echocardiography in the diagnosis of valvular perforations. American Journal of Cardiology. 2011;107(1):100–2.

[96] Bansal RC, Chandrasekaran K. Real time three-dimensional transesophageal echocardiographic evaluation of aortic valve perforation. Echocardiography. 2015;32(7):1147–56.

[97] Vijay SK, Tiwari BC, Misra M, Dwivedi SK. Incremental value of three-dimensional transthoracic echocardiography in the assessment of ruptured aneurysm of anterior mitral leaflet. Echocardiography. 2014;31(1):E24–E6.

[98] Walker N, Bhan A, Desai J, Monaghan MJ. Myocardial abscess: a rare complication of valvular endocarditis demonstrated by 3D contrast echocardiography. European Journal of Echocardiography: the Journal of the Working Group on Echocardiography of the European Society of Cardiology. 2010;11(10):E37–E.

[99] Naqvi TZ, Rafie R, Ghalichi M. Real-time 3D TEE for the diagnosis of right-sided endocarditis in patients with prosthetic devices. JACC: Cardiovascular Imaging. 2010;3(3):325–7.

[100] Jain R, Kolias TJ. Three-dimensional transesophageal echocardiography of pacemaker endocarditis. Journal of the American College of Cardiology. 2009;53(14):1241–.

[101] Sungur A, Hsiung MC, Meggo Quiroz LD, Oz TK, Haj Asaad A, Joshi D, et al. The advantages of live/real time three-dimensional transesophageal echocardiography in

the assessment of tricuspid valve infective endocarditis. Echocardiography. 2014;31(10): 1293–309.

[102] Tape TG, Panzer RJ. Echocardiography, endocarditis, and clinical information bias. Journal of General Internal Medicine. 1986;1(5):300–4.

[103] Stoddard MF, Liddell NE, Longaker RA, Dawkins PR. Transesophageal echocardiography: normal variants and mimickers. American Heart Journal. 1992;124(6):1587–98.

[104] Tornos P, Gonzalez-Alujas T, Thuny F, Habib G. Infective endocarditis: the European viewpoint. Current Problems in Cardiology. 2011;36(5):175–222.

[105] Rozich JD, Edwards WD, Hanna RD, Laffey DM, Johnson GH, Klarich KW. Mechanical prosthetic valve-associated strands: pathologic correlates to transesophageal echocardiography. Journal of the American Society of Echocardiography: Official Publication of the American Society of Echocardiography. 2003;16(1):97.

[106] Hill EE, Herijgers P, Claus P, Vanderschueren S, Peetermans WE, Herregods M-C. Clinical and echocardiographic risk factors for embolism and mortality in infective endocarditis. European Journal of Clinical Microbiology and Infectious Diseases. 2008;27(12):1159–64.

[107] Hubert S, Thuny F, Resseguier N, Giorgi R, Tribouilloy C, Le Dolley Y, et al. Prediction of symptomatic embolism in infective endocarditis. Journal of the American College of Cardiology. 2013;62(15):1384–92.

[108] Pamela S. Douglas, MD, FASE, Chair, Jeanne M. DeCara, MD, Richard B. Devereux, MD, Shelly Duckworth, RDCS, Julius M. Gardin, MD, FASE, Wael A. Jaber, MD, Annitta J. Morehead, RDCS, FASE, Jae K. Oh, MD, FASE, Michael H. Picard, MD, FASE, Scott D. Solomon, MD, Kevin Wei, MD, Neil J. Weissman, MD, FASE, Endorsed by the American College of Cardiology Foundation. Echocardiographic Imaging in Clinical Trials: American Society of Echocardiography Standards for Echocardiography Core Laboratories Journal of the American Society of Echocardiography. Durham, North Carolina; Chicago, Illinois; New York, New York; Hackensack, New Jersey; Cleveland, Ohio; Rochester, Minnesota; Boston, Massachusetts; Portland, Oregon; Washington, DC. 2009;22(7):755–765, DOI: http://dx.doi.org/10.1016/j.echo.2009.05.020.

[109] Chambers J, Sandoe J, Ray S, Prendergast B, Taggart D, Westaby S, et al. The infective endocarditis team: recommendations from an international working group. Heart 2014;100(7):524.

[110] Jaffe WM, Morgan DE, Pearlman AS, Otto CM. Infective endocarditis, 1983–1988: echocardiographic findings and factors influencing morbidity and mortality. Journal of the American College of Cardiology. 1990;15(6):1227–33.

[111] Thuny F, Di Salvo G, Belliard O, Avierinos JF, Pergola V, Rosenberg V, et al. Risk of embolism and death in infective endocarditis: prognostic value of echocardiography: a prospective multicenter study. [Erratum appears in Circulation. 2005 Aug

30;112(9):e125 Note: Disalvo, Giovanni [corrected to Di Salvo, Giovanni]; Calabro, Raffaello [corrected to Calabro, Raffaele]]. Circulation. 2005;112(1):69–75.

[112] Sanfilippo AJ, Picard MH, Newell JB, Rosas E, Davidoff R, Thomas JD, et al. Echocardiographic assessment of patients with infectious endocarditis: prediction of risk for complications. Journal of the American College of Cardiology. 1991;18(5):1191–9.

[113] Di Salvo G, Habib G, Pergola V, Avierinos J-F, Philip E, Casalta J-P, et al. Echocardiography predicts embolic events in infective endocarditis. Journal of the American College of Cardiology. 2001;37(4):1069–76.

[114] Vilacosta I, Graupner C, SanRomán J, Sarriá C, Ronderos R, Fernández C, et al. Risk of embolization after institution of antibiotic therapy for infective endocarditis. Journal of the American College of Cardiology. 2002;39(9):1489–95.

[115] San Román JA. Prognostic stratification of patients with left-sided endocarditis determined at admission. American Journal of Medicine. 2007;120(4):369.e1–.e7.

[116] Jassal DS, Neilan TG, Pradhan AD, Lynch KE, Vlahakes G, Agnihotri AK, et al. Surgical management of infective endocarditis: early predictors of short-term morbidity and mortality. The Annals of Thoracic Surgery. 2006;82(2):524–9.

[117] Lauridsen TK, Park L, Tong SYC, Selton-Suty C, Peterson G, Cecchi E, et al. Echocardiographic findings predict in-hospital and 1-year mortality in left-sided native valve staphylococcus aureus endocarditis: analysis from the international collaboration on endocarditis-prospective echo cohort study. Circulation: Cardiovascular Imaging. 2015;8(7):e003397.

[118] Bannay A, Hoen B, Duval X, Obadia J-F, Selton-Suty C, Le Moing V, et al. The impact of valve surgery on short- and long-term mortality in left-sided infective endocarditis: do differences in methodological approaches explain previous conflicting results? European Heart Journal. 2011;32(16):2003–15.

[119] Thuny F, Beurtheret S, Mancini J, Gariboldi V, Casalta J-P, Riberi A, et al. The timing of surgery influences mortality and morbidity in adults with severe complicated infective endocarditis: a propensity analysis. European Heart Journal. 2011;32(16):2027–33.

[120] Shapira Y, Weisenberg DE, Vaturi M, Sharoni E, Raanani E, Sahar G, et al. The impact of intraoperative transesophageal echocardiography in infective endocarditis. The Israel Medical Association Journal: IMAJ. 2007;9(4):299.

[121] Meagan M. Wasfy, Michael H. Picard. Transthoracic Echocardiography: nomenclature and standard views. In: Lang RM, Goldstein SA, Kronzon I, Khandheria B, Mor-Avi V, A B, editors. ASE's Comprehensive Echocardiography. 2nd. Philadelphia, PA: Elsevier; 2015. p. 19–45.

[122] Belham M. Transesophageal Echocardiography in Clinical Practice. London: Springer; 2009.

[123] Badano LP, Lang RM, Zamorano JL. Textbook of Real-time Three Dimensional Echocardiography. New York; London: Springer; 2011.

[124] Lang RM, Badano LP, Tsang W, Adams DH, Agricola E, Buck T, et al. EAE/ASE recommendations for image acquisition and display using three-dimensional echocardiography. Journal of the American Society of Echocardiography: Official Publication of the American Society of Echocardiography. 2012;25(1):3–46.

[125] Hahn RT, Abraham T, Adams MS, Bruce CJ, Glas KE, Lang RM, et al. Guidelines for performing a comprehensive transesophageal echocardiographic examination: recommendations from the American Society of Echocardiography and the Society of Cardiovascular Anesthesiologists. Journal of the American Society of Echocardiography: Official Publication of the American Society of Echocardiography. 2013;26(9):921–64.

[126] Mediratta A, Addetia K, Yamat M, Moss JD, Nayak HM, Burke MC, et al. 3D echocardiographic location of implantable device leads and mechanism of associated tricuspid regurgitation. JACC Cardiovascular Imaging 2014;7(4):337.

[127] Picard MH, American Society of E. American Society of Echocardiography Recommendations for Quality Echocardiography laboratory operations. Journal of the American Society of Echocardiography. 2011;24(1):1–10.

[128] Popescu BA, Andrade MJ, Badano LP, Fox KF, Flachskampf FA, Lancellotti P, et al. European Association of Echocardiography recommendations for training, competence, and quality improvement in echocardiography. European Journal of Echocardiography. 2009;10(8):893–905.

[129] Botelho-Nevers E, Thuny F, Casalta JP, Richet H, Gouriet F, Collart F, et al. Dramatic reduction in infective endocarditis–related mortality with a management-based approach. Archives of Internal Medicine. 2009;169(14):1290–8.

[130] Chirillo F, Scotton P, Rocco F, Rigoli R, Pedrocco A, Martire P, et al. Management strategies and outcome for prosthetic valve endocarditis. The American Journal of Cardiology. 2013;112(8):1177.

[131] Ali S, George LK, Das P, Koshy SKG. Intracardiac echocardiography: clinical utility and application. Echocardiography. 2011;28(5):582–90.

[132] Schwartz SL, Gillam LD, Weintraub AR, Sanzobrino BW, Hirst JA, Hsu T-L, et al. Intracardiac echocardiography in humans using a small-sized (6F), low frequency (12.5 MHz) ultrasound catheter methods, imaging planes and clinical experience. Journal of the American College of Cardiology. 1993;21(1):189–98.

[133] Ducas R, Tsang W, Chong AA, Jassal DS, Lang RM, Leong-Poi H, et al. Echocardiography and vascular ultrasound: new developments and future directions. Canadian Journal of Cardiology. 2013;29(3):304–16.

[134] Zucker EJ, Prabhakar AM, Ghoshhajra BB. The role of cardiac CT in the evaluation of endocarditis. Current Cardiovascular Imaging Reports. 2016;9(5):1–8.

[135] Grob A, Thuny F, Villacampa C, Flavian A, Gaubert JY, Raoult D, et al. Cardiac multidetector computed tomography in infective endocarditis: a pictorial essay. Insights into Imaging 2014;5(5):559–70.

[136] Thuny F, Gaubert J-Y, Jacquier A, Tessonnier L, Cammilleri S, Raoult D, et al. Imaging investigations in infective endocarditis: current approach and perspectives. Archives of Cardiovascular Diseases. 2013;106(1):52–62.

[137] Saby L, Laas O, Habib G, Cammilleri S, Mancini J, Tessonnier L, et al. Positron emission tomography/computed tomography for diagnosis of prosthetic valve endocarditis: increased valvular 18F-fluorodeoxyglucose uptake as a novel major criterion. Journal of the American College of Cardiology 2013;61(23):2374.

[138] Pizzi MN, Roque A, Fernández-Hidalgo N, Cuéllar-Calabria H, Ferreira-González I, Gonzàlez-Alujas MT, et al. Improving the diagnosis of infective endocarditis in prosthetic valves and intracardiac devices with 18F-fluordeoxyglucose positron emission tomography/computed tomography angiography: initial results at an infective endocarditis referral center. Circulation. 2015;132(12):1113–26.

[139] Dursun M, Yilmaz S, Yilmaz E, Yilmaz R, Onur I, Oflaz H, et al. The utility of cardiac MRI in diagnosis of infective endocarditis: preliminary results. Diagnostic and Interventional Radiology. 2015;21(1):28–33.

[140] Panizzi P, Stone JR, Nahrendorf M. Endocarditis and molecular imaging. Journal of nuclear cardiology: official publication of the American Society of Nuclear Cardiology. 2014;21(3):486–95.

Chapter 5

Ocular Manifestations of Endocarditis

Cheima Wathek and Riadh Rannen

Additional information is available at the end of the chapter

http://dx.doi.org/10.5772/65313

Abstract

Endocarditis is an inflammation of the inside lining of the heart chambers and heart valves. Ocular manifestations are nonspecific and could reveal the disease, justifying routine ocular examination. *Staphylococcus aureus* is the most incriminated in ocular complications. Endophthalmitis, retinal arterial occlusion, Roth dots, or vitreal and retinal infiltrations could be seen with endocarditis. Ocular prognosis in endophthalmitis and retinal arterial occlusion is poor. Ocular involvement was independently associated with death in infective endocarditis.

Keywords: endocarditis, eye, endophthalmitis, retinal arterial occlusion

1. Introduction

Ocular manifestations of endocarditis are nonspecific, caused by septic embolism and in rare cases by aseptic embolism. Ocular manifestations could reveal this disease. Routine ophthalmic examination should be considered for patients with infective endocarditis.

2. Epidemiology

There are no data presenting the epidemiology of ocular manifestations of endocarditis. However, many case reports reveal that ocular manifestations are common and could be the first manifestation of the disease. Roth dots are the most commonly seen in endocarditis. Other findings are described in case reports and include focal retinitis, embolic retinopathy, subretinal abscesses, choroidal septic metastasis, choroiditis, endophthalmitis, papillitis, and optic neuritis [1].

3. Physiopathology

Infective endocarditis, especially when associated with prosthetic cardiac valves, carries a very high complication rate. Among the most dreaded complications are perivalvular abscesses, intracardiac fistulae, acute heart failure (typically from acute aortic insufficiency—a very poorly tolerated physiologic condition), complete heart block, septic emboli, and pseudoaneurysms. In fact, embolic events occur in as many as 50% of all patients with infectious endocarditis. Specific organs and/or systems involved, from most to least common, include (A) central nervous system, 65%; (B) spleen, 20%; (C) hepatic, 14%; (D) renal, 14%; (E) musculoskeletal, 11%; and (F) mesenteric, 3% [1, 2].

4. Microbiology

Streptococcus is seen in over 58% of cases of infectious endocarditis. The most common germs seen in endophthalmitis and chorioretinitis are *Staphylococcus aureus*, *Staphylococcus epidermidis*, and *Streptococcus viridians*. *S. aureus* can lead to ocular complications in over 56% [3, 4]. Fungal endocarditis affects intravenous drug users and severe immunodeficiency patients (onco-hematology) [5]. *Candida* is the most common seen in fungal endocarditis.

5. Ocular clinical findings

5.1. Roth dots

A Roth dot is a cluster of superficial retinal hemorrhages ovally shaped, with pale center (**Figure 1**). It is commonly seen near the optic disk.

In endocarditis, this cluster represents red blood cells which surround inflammatory cells that have collected in the area in response to a septic embolism from valvular vegetations [1].

5.2. Retinal arterial occlusion

Retinal arterial occlusion occurs as a complication of septic or aseptic embolism. Clinical manifestations depend on the localization of occlusion. We distinguish the following.

5.2.1. Central retinal arterial occlusion

Patient, if conscious, presents sudden, complete, and painless loss of vision in one eye. Fundoscopy shows pale edema of the retina, particularly in the posterior pole where the nerve fiber and ganglion cell layers are thickest. The orange reflex of the foveola with intact choroidal vasculature contrasts with the surrounding opaque neural retina, producing the cherry red spot. Central retinal arterial occlusion (CRAO) has a poor prognosis. If not treated in the first hour, it can lead to permanent loss of vision and other ocular complications [6].

http://dx.doi.org/10.5772/65313

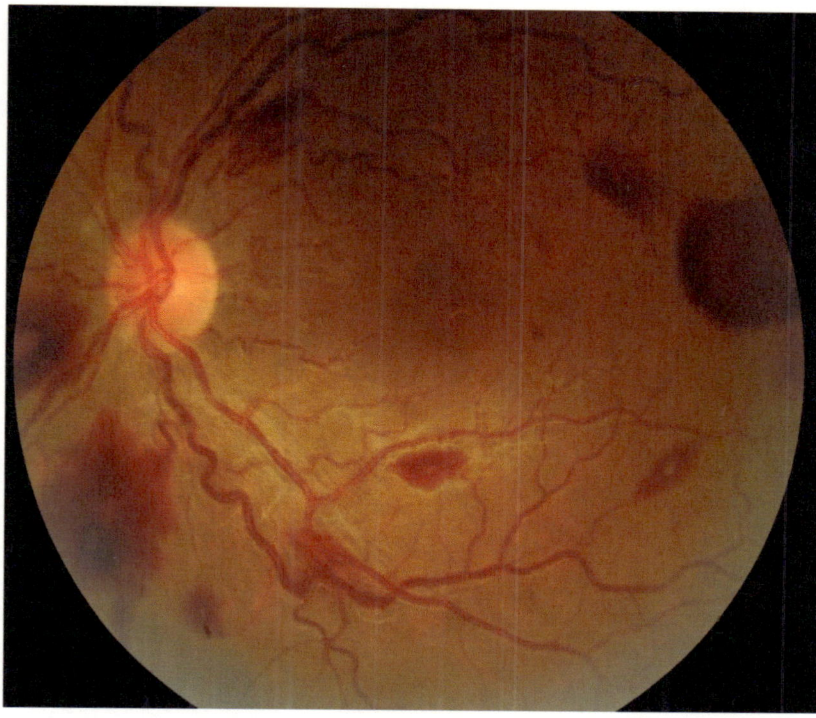

Figure 1. Fundoscopy of the left eye showing multiple Roth dots.

5.2.2. Branch retinal arterial occlusion

Branch retinal arterial occlusion (BRAO) may be clinically asymptomatic. If symptomatic, patient may report a loss of vision or visual field amputation. Fundoscopy shows a pale edema due to infarction of the inner retina in the distribution of the affected vessel. With time, the occluded vessel recanalizes, perfusion returns, and the edema resolves; however, a permanent field defect remains.

5.2.3. Ophthalmic arterial occlusion

This event is responsible for an interruption of both retinal and posterior ciliary circulations. The visual prognosis, in this entity, is usually worse. If conscious, patient presents pain, sudden and complete loss of vision. Ophthalmic examination revealed no light perception, ophthalmoplegia (**Figure 2**), and nonreactive mydriasis. Fundoscopy showed remarkable edema of the entire retina, resulting from inner and outer retinal ischemia and whitened retinal vessels (**Figure 3**). The cherry-red spot is not noted in this case because of choroidal compromise and probable retinal pigment epithelial or choroidal opacification, or both, in about 40% of eyes. Fluorescein angiography revealed impairment of retinal vascular and choroidal flows (**Figure 4**). A cherry-red spot may be initially absent, but then appear over a several-day period as choroid perfusion improves [7].

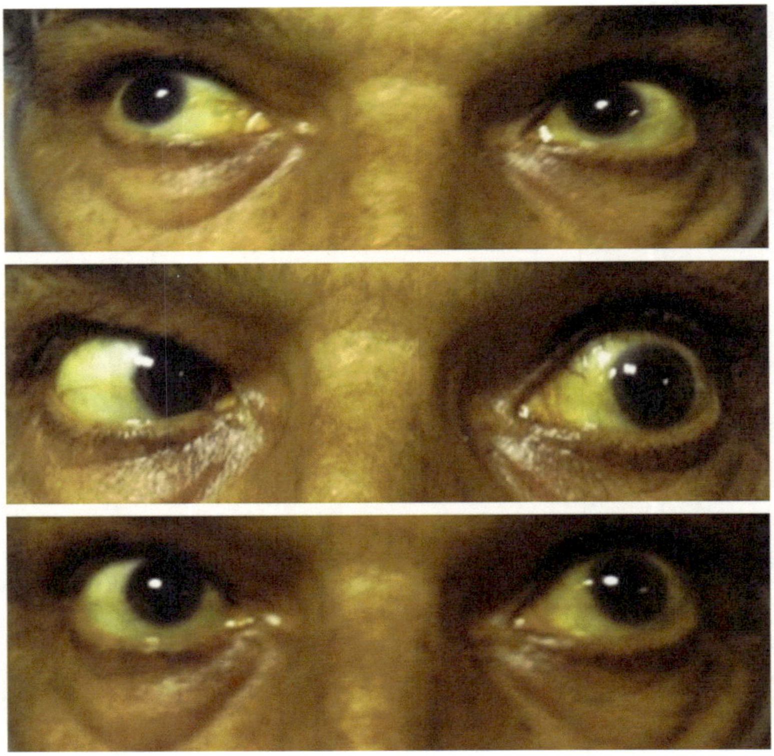

Figure 2. Ophthalmoplegia of the left eye.

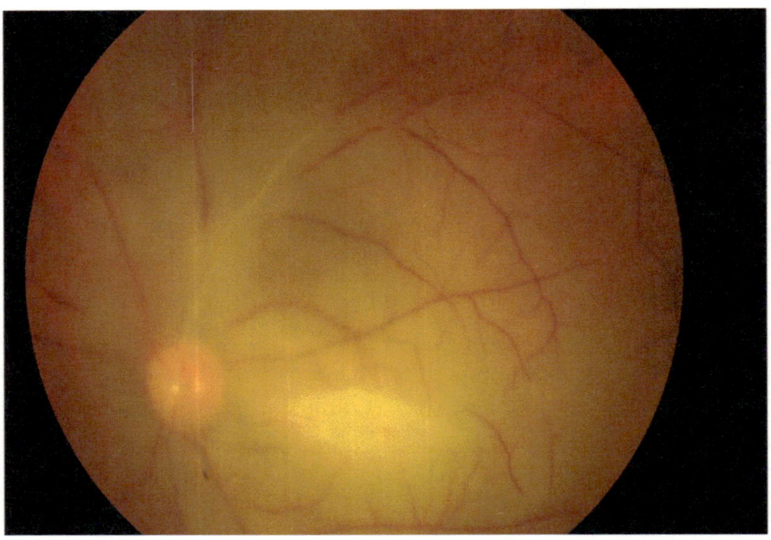

Figure 3. Fundus photograph showing edema of the entire left retina and whitened retinal vessels without cherry-red spot.

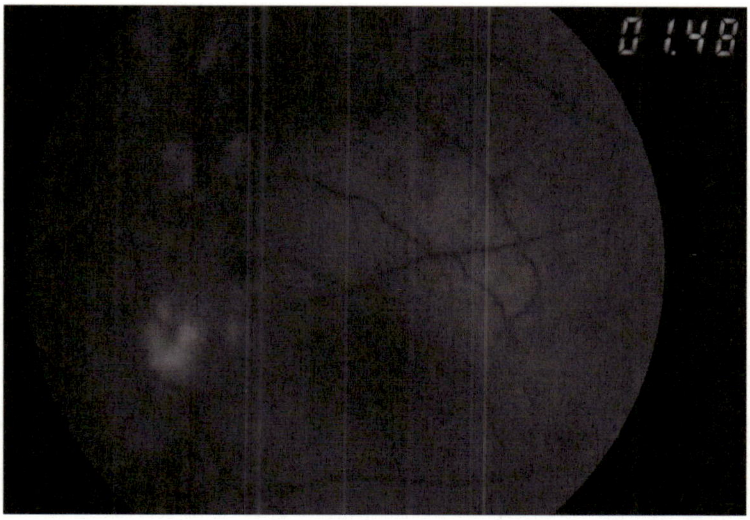

Figure 4. Fluorescein angiography showing late onset of choroidal perfusion and nonopacification of both retinal artery and vein.

5.3. Retinal and vitreal infiltration

Septic embolism can lead to posterior uveitis (retinitis, chorioretinitis, choroiditis, and vitreal infiltration). In most cases, posterior uveitis is misdiagnosed and is complicated by endophthalmitis (**Figure 5**).

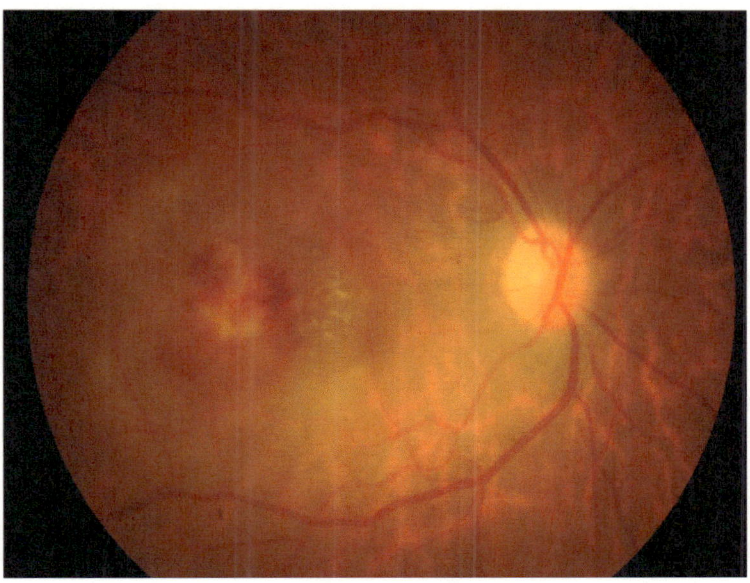

Figure 5. Fundoscopy showing retinal and vitreous infiltrations in bacterial endocarditis.

5.4. Endophthalmitis

Endophthalmitis is a condition when all the internal structures of the eye are invaded with replicating microorganisms and associated with an important inflammatory response.

Endogenous bacterial endophthalmitis is a rare pathology that affects individuals of any age and represents 2–15% of all cases. Endocarditis is the second more frequent cause of endogenous endophthalmitis after meningitis.

The rate of endophthalmitis can raise 50% with endocarditis to *S. aureus*. The right eye is generally more affected than the left eye.

The onset of the signs and symptoms depends on the pathogenic virulence. Typically, patient presents pain, chemosis, proptosis, hypopyon, and corneal melting.

Blood culture findings are positive in more than 90% of infective endocarditis cases. The most common etiological germ is *Streptococcus* 45.7% and the valvular was affected in 27.2% of the episodes. Systemic therapy may be sufficient when the vitreous cavity is not greatly involved. In the other cases, antibiotic intravitreal injections and vitrectomy are necessary [5, 8–11].

5.5. Choroidal neovascularization

Subretinal neovascularization secondary to choroidal septic metastasis was reported in two cases. Neovascularization occurs in choroidal scars with variable delay (10 months and 5 years) [12].

6. Prognosis

Ocular prognosis depends on the ocular manifestation. Functional prognosis of retinal arterial occlusion and endophthalmitis is bad in most cases. Ocular involvement was independently associated with death in infective endocarditis.

Author details

Cheima Wathek* and Riadh Rannen

*Address all correspondence to: wcheima@yahoo.fr

Military Hospital of Tunis, Ophthalmology Department, Faculty of Medicine of Tunis, Tunis El Manar University, Tunis, Tunisia

References

[1] Klig JE. Ophthalmologic complications of systemic disease. Emerg Med Clin N Am 2008;26:217–31.

[2] Gergaud JM, Breux JP, Grollier G, Roblot P, Becq-Giraudon B. Current aspects of infectious endocarditis: apropos of 53 cases. Ann Med Interne 1994;145(3): 163–7.

[3] Mainardi L. Bactériologie. Masson 2ème Edition 2011:117–18.

[4] Jung J, Lee J, Yu SN, Kim YK, Lee JY, Sung H et al. Incidence and risk factors of ocular infection caused by *Staphylococcus aureus* bacteremia. Antimicrob Agents Chemother 2016;60(4):2012–7.

[5] Silva-Vergara ML, de Camargo ZP, Silva PF, Abdalla MR, Sgarbieri RN, et al. Case report: disseminated *Sporothrix brasiliensis* infection with endocardial and ocular involvement in an HIV-infected patient. Am J Trop Med Hyg 2012;86(3):477–80.

[6] Liliana M, Pitta ML, Peresa M, Ferreirab V, Pugab MC, Severinoa D, da Silva GF. Retinal artery embolization complicating Libman-Sacks endocarditis in a systemic lupus erythematosus patient. Rev Port Cardiol 2013;32(4):345–7.

[7] Wathek C, Kharrat O, Maalej A, Nafaa MF, Rannen R, Gabsi S. Ophthalmic artery occlusion as a complication of infectious endocarditis. J Fr Ophthalmol 2014;37(10):e161–3.

[8] Zayit-Soudry S, Neudorfer M, Barak A, et al. Endogenous *Phialemonium curvatum* endophthalmitis. Am J Ophthalmol 2005;140(4):755–7.

[9] Arcieri ES, Jorge EF, de Abrea Ferreira L, et al. Bilateral endogenous endophthalmitis associated with infective endocarditis: case report. Braz J Infect Dis 2001;5(6):356–9.

[10] Shmuely H, Kremer I, Sagie A, et al. Candida tropicalis multifocal endophthalmitis as the only initial manifestation of pacemaker endocarditis. Am J Ophthalmol 1997;123(4): 559–60.

[11] Verweij PE, Rademakers AJ, Koopmans PP, et al. Endophthalmitis as presenting symptoms of group G streptococcal endocarditis. Infection 1994;22(1):56–7.

[12] Munier F, Othenin-Girard P. Subretinal neovascularization secondary to choroidal septic metastasis from acute bacterial endocarditis. Retina 1992;12:108–12.

Chapter 6

Culture Negative Endocarditis: Advances in Diagnosis and Treatment

Marion J. Skalweit

Additional information is available at the end of the chapter

http://dx.doi.org/10.5772/64920

Abstract

Culture-negative endocarditis (CNE) is a challenging clinical entity, both diagnostically and therapeutically. In this chapter, the changed epidemiology and microbiology of CNE are reviewed with cases highlighting typical pathogens in patients pre-treated with antibiotics, less common fastidious pathogens such as bacteria of the HACEK group, nutritionally deficient bacteria, *Legionella* spp. and Mycobacteria, "quintessential" CNE pathogens such as *Bartonella* spp., *Coxiella burnetti* and *Tropheryma* whipplei, as well as fungal CNE. Contemporary diagnostic methods are reviewed including polymerase chain reaction-based pathogen 16s RNA amplification coupled with electrospray ionization mass spectrometry (PCR/ESI-MS). Finally, treatment options per the recently updated 2015 American Heart Association and European Society for Cardiology guideline are presented.

Keywords: culture-negative endocarditis, *Bartonella* spp., *Coxiella burnetti* and *Tropheryma whipplei*, PCR/ESI-MS

1. Introduction

Culture-negative endocarditis (CNE) is one of the most challenging infectious diseases clinical syndromes both diagnostically and therapeutically. The prevalence of CNE varies widely in various modern series: it is estimated that on average, in 20% (range 5–71%) of echocardiographically evident endocarditis, both native and prosthetic valve, blood cultures do not yield a specific pathogen [1–7]. The morbidity but not necessarily mortality associated with CNE is higher than in instances where a specific pathogen is found, primarily due to the increased burden of diagnostic testing, delays in administration of antibiotics and the extended use of broad spectrum anti-microbial agents [8]. This chapter will review the epidemiology and likely microbiology of CNE, as well as enhanced diagnostic methods and treatment recommendations.

A useful definition of CNE has been put forth by Tattevin et al. [9] wherein one can think of this entity as (1) true bacterial endocarditis with blood cultures sterilized by previous receipt of antimicrobials; (2) CNE caused by fastidious or unusual organisms such as the bacteria known as the "HACEK" group, nutritionally deficient *Streptococci, Pasturella* spp., *Helicobacter* spp., Mycobacteria and fungal organisms and (3) "true" CNE involving intracellular organisms that are detectable via serology or polymerase chain reaction (PCR) of valvular tissue, e.g. *Bartonella quintana, Coxiella burnetti* and *Tropheryma whipplei*. In addition, there are non-infectious causes of endocarditis, e.g. murantic that will not be covered in this chapter.

2. Epidemiology of CNE

The epidemiology of infective endocarditis, and hence CNE, has changed over the last five decades [5, 10]. Patients are generally older and male, with greater numbers of hospital associated cases, and with indwelling devices such as catheters, pacemakers and prosthetic valves. Accordingly the numbers of cases of infective endocarditis with *Staphylococcus aureus*, coagulase-negative *Staphylococci* and *Enterococci* have increased. With the advent of novel diagnostic methods (PCR-based testing), the prevalence of CNE may have decreased to 14.2% [5] in the last decade, but other reviews indicate otherwise [10]. Specific aspects of the patient's medical history may provide "epidemiological clues" (Table 6 in Ref. [1]) to the microbiological cause. Military personnel have some higher risk of CNE due to *C. burnetti* for example [11].

3. Microbiology of CNE

The microbiology of CNE is varied and depends on host and environmental factors that predispose to one type of pathogen versus another [1]. As per the classification of Tattevin et al. [9], the microbiologic discussion will follow this paradigm.

3.1. CNE due to pre-treatment of typical bacterial endocarditis

According to one of the largest surveys of infective endocarditis recently performed, in the last decade, 29.7% of IE were due to *S. aureus*, 17.6% were due to oral *Streptococci*, 10% were due to coagulase-negative *Staphylococci* and 10% were due to *Enterococci*. Approximately, 16% of IE cases were thus due to Gram-negative bacteria, fungi and mycobacteria that could be cultured from blood. Because the presentation of infective endocarditis can be non-specific and is often associated with clinical sepsis, patients receive empiric broad spectrum anti-bacterials before sufficient numbers of blood cultures can be obtained. In one contemporary survey, antibiotics were used before blood cultures 74% of the time, with many patients coming from outside hospitals before a diagnosis of endocarditis was established [4]. The distribution of bacterial etiologies in these cases should represent what is seen generally when blood cultures are obtained prior to initiation of antibiotics. PCR of valve tissue in the cases where pretreatment occurred showed a predominance of *Streptococcus oralis* (54%), *Streptococcus aureus* (7.7%) and *Streptococcus gallolyticus* (formerly known as *Streptococcus bovis*) 5.1%. This likely reflects the ability of these organisms to attach to endovascular epithelium and be detectable by PCR methods.

3.2. CNE due to fastidious micro-organisms

3.2.1. HACEK group

Much of the early literature regarding CNE focused on infections with so-called "fastidious" organisms that were traditionally difficult to grow in blood culture, due to specific nutritional requirements of these organisms. These included a number of oral Gram-negative bacteria (*Haemophilus* species, *Aggregatibacter* species, *Cardiobacterium hominis, Eikenella corrodens* and *Kingella* species) that came to be known by the acronym "HACEK" (reviewed in [12]). Automated blood culture methodology involved the use of media that lacked particular nutrients like hemin, and extended incubation of 3 weeks was recommended in order to isolate HACEK group and other fastidious Gram negatives (ref). However, as early as 1993, it was evident that extended incubation was no longer necessary in order to isolate these bacteria [13, 14]. Standard 5–7 day incubation was sufficient to recover an organism in most instances.

HACEK organisms are rarely the cause of infective endocarditis, and because of the improved ability to isolate these organisms from standard blood culture specimens, even more rarely the cause of CNE. In a recent series, four out of 77 patients with HACEK IE had negative blood cultures [15]. Of these, three had previously received antibiotics. Diagnosis was made by culture of devices, and in one patient, by PCR of valvular tissue. *Cardiobacterium valvarum* has been described as an unusual *Cardiobacterium* spp. associated with endocarditis, in this case, an infected aortic graft in a middle-aged man with gingivitis and a sub-acute bacterial endocarditis presentation. In this case, the organism grew in blood culture but could not be identified by routine microbiological examination. 16S rRNA analysis revealed the species.

Pediatric populations, especially young children between the ages of 6 months and four years, appear to be particularly vulnerable to infections with *Kingella kingae* [16]. *K. kingae* is present in the oropharynx and respiratory tract of young children and can be transmitted person-to-person with resulting outbreaks of infection. *K. kingae* has a variety of colonization and virulence factors such as pili that allows the organism to anchor itself to human mucosal epithelium, polysaccharide capsule that decreases opsonization by complement, the ability to produce exopolysaccharide and biofilm that is an important factor in the formation of endovascular vegetations and RTX toxin, a potent cytotoxin that targets macrophages and respiratory epithelium [17]. Fortunately, bacteremia and endocarditis are relatively rare syndromes associated with this organism [16], causing 7.1–7.8% of pediatric endocarditis cases [18, 19]. The presentation can be dramatic as illustrated in a child with mycotic aneurysm of the aorta and cerebral infarcts [20].

3.2.2. *Non HACEK group organisms*

Other fastidious bacteria causing CNE include *Pasturella multocida* and other *Pasturella* spp. which constitute part of the normal oral flora of dogs and cats in particular [21]. While bite wounds are obviously a portal of entry for *Pasturella* spp., in immunocompromised patients, more superficial contact especially with cat fur, minor cat scratches and cat saliva can lead to bacteremia and subsequent endocarditis [22]. Culture-negative endocarditis caused by *Abiotrophia defectiva* and *Granulicatella* spp.—so-called nutritionally deficient *Streptococci* [23] —can also be associated with infected intracranial aneurysms and may be difficult to isolate in routine blood cultures [24]. Special consideration for length of therapy must be given and is covered below. *Clostridia* and other anaerobic organisms [25] may be difficult to recover in routine blood cultures if specimens are not handled appropriately. These organisms are likely a rare cause of CNE, but true prevalence is unknown. *Gemella* spp. have been described rarely as a cause of CNE [9, 21] including *Gemella burgeri* tricuspid valve endocarditis [26] and *Gemella hemolysans* prosthetic valve endocarditits identified by PCR of prosthetic valve material and requiring implantation of a total artificial heart as a bridge to transplantation [27]. *Brucella mellitensis* is another unusual pathogen associated with culture-negative endocarditis [2], especially in regions of the world where consumption of unpasteurized milk (cow, goat and sheep) occurs. In one series of six patients subsequently found to have *Brucella* endocarditis, only two patients had blood cultures that revealed the diagnosis [28]. Several different *Legionella* spp. have been reported as causes of culture-negative endocarditis, both in native valves and prosthetic valves. These include cases of *Legionella pneumophila* in an immunocompromised patient with pneumonitis, a positive BAL fluid *Legionella* antigen, and subsequent BAL fluid and blood isolation of the organism when subcultured onto buffered charcoal yeast extract agar (BCYE agar) [29]. Another CNE case with *L. pneumophila* was identified when the patient presented with septic arthritis and the organism was identified from synovial fluid by 16s rDNA PCR and was subsequently found to have a new murmur and a mitral vegetation [30]. Mycobacteria are another rare cause of CNE, especially in association with porcine bioprosthetic valves [31]. This study from a reference laboratory conducted between 2010 and 2013 found PCR evidence of Mycobacterial infection in six out of 370 valve samples submitted from patients with suspected CN [31] with five cases of *Mycobacterium chelonae* and one case of *M. lentiflavum****. While typically associated with immunodeficiency states, mycobacterial infections have also been reported in immunocompetent hosts as in the case of a patient with disseminated *M. chelonae* infection and resulting pacemaker CNE [32]. Special stains and cultures for acid fast bacilli should be considered in patients with device-related CNE [33]. Finally there are also rare reports with unusual causes of endovascular infections such as CNE in an immunocompromised patient on high dose corticosteroids [34] and infected aortic aneurysm in an immunocompetent patient [35] with *Helicobacter cinaedi*.

3.3. CNE due to *Bartonella* spp., *C. burnetti* and *T. whipplei*

This section deals with CNE attributable to organisms that are not typically identified with blood cultures but are responsible for a significant portion of cases of culture-negative infective endocarditis [36].

Bartonella endocarditis has been described as the "quintessential culture-negative endocarditis" [37]. *Bartonella* species were first described as a cause of infectious endocarditis in 1993 (reviewed in [38]). A recent study in Brazil estimated that 19.6% of CNE cases were due to *Bartonella* spp. [36]. There are currently 23 different species of *Bartonella* reported; the most common etiology of CNE, however, is the result of louse transmitted *B. quintana* especially in homeless persons, or infection with *Bartonella henselae* transmitted by contact with young cats. *B. henselae* is more often associated with immunocompromised hosts and prosthetic valve endocarditis [39–41]. Diagnosis of *Bartonella* CNE is typically made via serologies and/or PCR of valvular material. Further modifications to the modified Duke diagnostic criteria for endocarditis have been proposed to incorporate positive PCR, Western blot or serum IgG titer ≥800 as major criteria [38]. Unusual clinical presentations with severe renal impairment have been described with *Bartonella* CNE where there is a delay in diagnosis including anti-neutrophil cytoplasmic antibody (ANCA) positive necrotizing glomerulonephritis [42], C3 predominant glomerulonephritis [39] and proliferative glomerulonephritis (GN) with erythroblastopenia [43]. One case of *B. henselae* tricuspid valve CNE was diagnosed after the patient presented with chronic pulmonary emboli [44]. In this patient, the source was felt to be a tick bite rather than exposure to cats.

C. burnetti is a rickettsial like organism associated with true CNE [9, 21]. In Brazil, it was estimated that the prevalence of *C. burnetti* as a cause of CNE was 7.9% [36] by PCR and serologic methods. In France, in the 1990s, annual incidence was estimated at 1 per million or <5% of all cases of endocarditis [45]. Acquisition in humans is usually through exposure to parturient animals such as sheep [21]. Presentation can be quite severe especially in immunocompromised persons, pregnant women and in persons with prosthetic valves or native valvular heart disease [46]. A new genotype, MST 54 [47] was recently described in a child with CNE secondary to congenital heart disease from an area endemic for *C. burnetti*.

T. whipplei is an *Actinomycete* bacterium found in the stool and environment [48]. Stool carriage in uninfected humans can be detected in the range of wards of 4–31%. An infectious cause of lipodystrophia intestinalis, later known as Whipple's disease, was first proposed by George Whipple in 1907 based on the presence of lipid laden foamy macrophages in the lamina propria of the small intestine. Clinical manifestations are protean, but generally patients present with diarrhea, weight loss, fever and malabsorption. *T. whipplei* is a known cause of CNE, and its true prevalence may be underestimated. When associated with arthralgia in middle-age men, it is almost pathognomonic for *T. whipplei* as the etiologic agent [49, 50]. While the organism can be cultured in fibroblasts [48], diagnosis of CNE typically requires PCR analysis of valvular tissue [51].

3.4. CNE due to fungal pathogens

Invasive mold infections are another cause of CNE, due to the difficulty in isolating these organisms from routine blood cultures. They are an important cause especially of early culture-negative prosthetic valve endocarditis [52] but can cause late prosethetic valve, pacemaker associated as well as native valve endocarditis. Among cases in the recent literature, infections with *Aspergillus* spp. [53–55], *Histoplasma capsulatum* [56–58] and *Trichosporin* spp. [59,

60] are the most widely reported. Commercial tests that detect fungal wall antigens such as galactomannan [2, 61, 62] and β-1,3-D-glucan [62] can show good sensitivity and specificity in diagnosis of fungal CNE. Jinno et al. [56] reported negative urine *Histoplasma* antigen results in their patient with *H. capsulatum* CNE, with diagnosis based on valvular pathology and tissue culture.

4. Diagnostic methods

Our understanding of the etiology of CNE and our ability to offer more targeted treatment to patients with CNE have been dramatically affected by the large number of novel diagnostic tests now available to add to our investigative armamentarium. The following discussion will focus on methods that allow diagnosis without removal of infected valves or cardiac devices (prosthetic valves, endovascular grafts, pacemaker and defibrillator leads, ventricular assist devices, etc.) versus methods that require removal of tissue or a device for diagnostic and therapeutic reasons.

4.1. Non-invasive methods

Imaging using positron emission tomography (PET) scanning has been utilized to diagnose a case of *T. whipplei* endocarditis [63]. The infected prosthetic valve was subsequently removed providing material for PCR-based methods to confirm the diagnosis, but the impetus to remove the valve came from the PET scan. Four-dimensional cardiac MRI was used to better define valvular damage and diagnose aortic valve endocarditis in a case of *C. burnetti* CNE in a patient with exposure to domesticated buffalos and positive serologies [64]. PCR combined with electrospray ionization mass spectrometry (PCR/ESI-MS) methods have been applied to detect pathogens in blood cultures in patients already receiving antibiotics and made a diagnosis in 41 out of 410 cases, although not specifically in persons with CNE [65]. Broad range PCR on blood culture specimens has also been utilized [2]. Serum galactomannan and β-1,3-D-glucan have already been mentioned as serum diagnostic tests for fungal CNE [2, 61, 62].

4.2. Invasive methods

Methodologies to increase numbers of planktonic organisms that can be cultured from devices have been devised, using sonication of the devices [66, 67]. Metagenomic analysis of the results of next generation sequencing has been used to diagnose *A. defectiva* CNE [68]. A universal PCR/sequencing test has been applied to diagnose CNE on blood and valvular tissue [69]. Immunofluorescent antibody detection, Western blot analysis and real time-PCR of 16s RNA have been used to diagnose CNE due to *Bartonella* spp. [38]. PCR/ESI-MS has been utilized on valve tissue to diagnose CNE [70, 71].

5. Treatment of CNE

There are some distinct differences in the management of infective endocarditis according to the United States [1] versus European guidelines [72] updated in 2015. These are reviewed in Tattevin et al. [73]. However, in regard to treatment of the following etiologic agents of CNE, there is good agreement in general.

5.1. Empiric therapy for CNE

For patients with acute clinical presentations of native valve endocarditis, according to the US guidelines, empiric coverage for *S. aureus*, β-hemolytic *Streptococci* and aerobic Gram-negative bacilli is provided. Such regimens should include vancomycin and cefepime at the beginning. For patients with a subacute presentation of native valve endocarditis, additional empirical coverage of viridans *Streptococci*, HACEK and *Enterococci* is added. Vancomycin and ampicillin-sulbactam is a suggested regimen. If blood cultures eventually become positive for a typical pathogen, empiric treatment can be tailored accordingly. For patients with early (<1 year) culture-negative prosthetic valve endocarditis, empiric coverage for *Staphylococci, Streptococci, Enterococci* and Gram-negative bacilli is appropriate. Vancomycin, rifampin, gentamicin and cefepime are offered as options. For late prosthetic valve endocarditis, antibiotic therapy to cover viridans *Streptococci, Staphylococci* and *Enterococci* such as vancomycin and ceftriaxone is suggested. Empiric antibiotics can be narrowed based on specific pathogens that are subsequently identified. Surgical source control and removal of infected devices are required more often with the pathogens associated with CNE.

5.2. *A. defectiva, Granulicatella* spp.

As summarized in the European guidelines, these nutritionally deficient bacteria produce endocarditis with a protracted course which is associated with large vegetations (≥10 mm), higher rates of complications and valve replacement (around 50%), possibly due to delayed diagnosis and treatment. Antibiotic recommendations include penicillin G, ceftriaxone or vancomycin for 6 weeks, combined with an aminoglycoside for at least the first 2 weeks.

6. HACEK

Per the US and European guidelines, microbiologic susceptibility testing might be difficult to perform on HACEK microorganisms, and they should be considered ampicillin resistant secondary to β-lactamase production. Penicillin and ampicillin should not be used for the treatment of patients with endocarditis. Ceftriaxone should be used unless the patient has a severe β-lactam allergy. The duration of therapy for HACEK native valve endocarditis is 4 weeks; for prosthetic valve infections, duration of therapy is 6 weeks or longer. Gentamicin is not recommended in the US guidelines because of its nephrotoxicity risks but is an option in the European guidelines. A fluoroquinolone (ciprofloxacin, levofloxacin, ormoxifloxacin) can be used in patients with a β-lactam allergy. Ampicillin-sulbactam is also a treatment option.

Bartonella spp.	Doxycycline 100 mg/12 h orally for 4 weeks plus gentamicin (3 mg/24 h) i.v. for 2 weeks
Brucella spp.	Doxycycline (200 mg/24 h) plus cotrimoxazole (960 mg/12 h) plus rifampin (300–600/24 h) for ≥3–6 months orally
Coxiella burnetti	Doxycycline (200 mg/24 h) plus hydroxychloroquine (200–600 mg/24 h) orally (>18 months of treatment)
Legionella spp.	Levofloxacin (500 mg/12 h) i.v. or orally for ≥6 weeks or clarithromycin (500 mg/12 h) i.v. for 2 weeks, then orally for 4 weeks plus rifampin (300–1200 mg/24 h)
T. whipplei	Doxycycline (200 mg/24 h) plus hydroxychloroquine (200–600 mg/24 h)c orally for ≥18 months

Treatment of the following unusual pathogens in CNE is best summarized in the European guidelines and in Broqui et al. [21].

7. Fungal CNE

Per the European guidelines, for *Aspergillus* infections, voriconazole is the drug of choice, and some experts recommend the addition of an echinocandin or amphotericin B. Surgery is generally required, and prolonged suppressive therapy is recommended. For *H. capsulatum*, surgical management followed by 6 weeks of amphotericin B and additional suppressive oral itraconazole is recommended. Most agents have poor activity against other mold species like *Trichosporon* spp. The mainstay of therapy is surgical.

Author details

Marion J. Skalweit

Address all correspondence to: msh5@case.edu

Louis Stokes Cleveland Department of Veterans Affairs Medical Center and Case Western Reserve University School of Medicine, Departments of Medicine and Biochemistry, Division of Infectious Diseases, Ohio, USA

References

[1] Baddour LM, Wilson WR, Bayer AS, Fowler VG, Jr., Tleyjeh IM, Rybak MJ, et al. Infective endocarditis in adults: diagnosis, antimicrobial therapy, and management of complications: a scientific statement for healthcare professionals from the American Heart Association. Circulation. 2015 Oct 13;132(15):1435–86. PubMed PMID: 26373316.

[2] El-Kholy AA, El-Rachidi NG, El-Enany MG, AbdulRahman EM, Mohamed RM, Rizk HH. Impact of serology and molecular methods on improving the microbiologic diagnosis of infective endocarditis in Egypt. Infection. 2015 Oct;43(5):523–9. PubMed PMID: 25808262.

[3] Hase R, Otsuka Y, Yoshida K, Hosokawa N. Profile of infective endocarditis at a tertiary-care hospital in Japan over a 14-year period: characteristics, outcome and predictors for in-hospital mortality. Int J Infect Dis. 2015 Apr;33:62–6. PubMed PMID: 25576825.

[4] Lamas CC, Fournier PE, Zappa M, Brandao TJ, Januario-da-Silva CA, Correia MG, et al. Diagnosis of blood culture-negative endocarditis and clinical comparison between blood culture-negative and blood culture-positive cases. Infection. 2015 Dec 15 44(4): 459–66. PubMed PMID: 26670038.

[5] Slipczuk L, Codolosa JN, Davila CD, Romero-Corral A, Yun J, Pressman GS, et al. Infective endocarditis epidemiology over five decades: a systematic review. PLoS One. 2013;8(12):e82665. PubMed PMID: 24349331. Pubmed Central PMCID: 3857279.

[6] Topan A, Carstina D, Slavcovici A, Rancea R, Capalneanu R, Lupse M. Assesment of the Duke criteria for the diagnosis of infective endocarditis after twenty-years. An analysis of 241 cases. Clujul Med. 2015;88(3):321–6. PubMed PMID: 26609264. Pubmed Central PMCID: 4632890.

[7] Wang LW, Noel B, Descloux E, Baron DW. Antiphospholipid syndrome: an important differential diagnosis for culture-negative endocarditis. Am J Med. 2015 Mar;128(3): 250–3. PubMed PMID: 25433300.

[8] Siciliano RF, Mansur AJ, Castelli JB, Arias V, Grinberg M, Levison ME, et al. Community-acquired culture-negative endocarditis: clinical characteristics and risk factors for mortality. Int J Infect Dis. 2014 Aug;25:191–5. PubMed PMID: 24971520.

[9] Tattevin P, Watt G, Revest M, Arvieux C, Fournier PE. Update on blood culture-negative endocarditis. Med Mal Infect. 2015 Jan–Feb;45(1–2):1–8. PubMed PMID: 25480453.

[10] Vogkou CT, Vlachogiannis NI, Palaiodimos L, Kousoulis AA. The causative agents in infective endocarditis: a systematic review comprising 33,214 cases. European Journal of Clinical Microbiology & Infectious Diseases: Official Publication of the European Society of Clinical Microbiology. 2016 May 11 35(8):1227–45. PubMed PMID: 27170145.

[11] Gough A, Clay K, Williams A, Jackson S, Prendergast B. Infective endocarditis in the military patient. J R Army Med Corps. 2015 Sep;161(3):283–7. PubMed PMID: 26243804.

[12] Revest M, Egmann G, Cattoir V, Tattevin P. HACEK endocarditis: state-of-the-art. Expert Rev Anti Infect Ther. 2016 May;14(5):523–30. PubMed PMID: 26953488.

[13] Baron EJ, Scott JD, Tompkins LS. Prolonged incubation and extensive subculturing do not increase recovery of clinically significant microorganisms from standard automated blood cultures. Clin Infect Dis. 2005 Dec 1;41(11):1677–80. PubMed PMID: 16267743.

[14] Doern GV, Davaro R, George M, Campognone P. Lack of requirement for prolonged incubation of Septi-Chek blood culture bottles in patients with bacteremia due to fastidious bacteria. Diagn Microbiol Infect Dis. 1996 Mar;24(3):141–3. PubMed PMID: 8724399.

[15] Chambers ST, Murdoch D, Morris A, Holland D, Pappas P, Almela M, et al. HACEK infective endocarditis: characteristics and outcomes from a large, multi-national cohort. PLoS One. 2013;8(5):e63181. PubMed PMID: 23690995. Pubmed Central PMCID: 3656887.

[16] Principi N, Esposito S. *Kingella kingae* infections in children. BMC infectious diseases. 2015;15:260. PubMed PMID: 26148872. Pubmed Central PMCID: 4494779.

[17] Yagupsky P. Kingella kingae: carriage, transmission, and disease. Clin Microbiol Rev. 2015 Jan;28(1):54–79. PubMed PMID: 25567222. Pubmed Central PMCID: 4284298.

[18] Marom D, Levy I, Gutwein O, Birk E, Ashkenazi S. Healthcare-associated versus community-associated infective endocarditis in children. The Pediatric infectious disease journal. 2011 Jul;30(7):585–8. PubMed PMID: 21289530.

[19] Webb R, Voss L, Roberts S, Hornung T, Rumball E, Lennon D. Infective endocarditis in New Zealand children 1994–2012. The Pediatric infectious disease journal. 2014 May; 33(5):437–42. PubMed PMID: 24378941.

[20] Feldman LF, Hersh Z, Birk E, Amir G, Wertheimer G. [Mycotic aneurysm of the ascending aorta and cerebral infarcts in a 17-month old child with *Kingella kingae* endocarditis]. Harefuah. 2015 Jun;154(6):369–72, 405. PubMed PMID: 26281080.

[21] Brouqui P, Raoult D. Endocarditis due to rare and fastidious bacteria. Clin Microbiol Rev. 2001 Jan;14(1):177–207. PubMed PMID: 11148009. Pubmed Central PMCID: 88969.

[22] Wilkie IW, Harper M, Boyce JD, Adler B. *Pasteurella multocida*: diseases and pathogenesis. Curr Top Microbiol Immunol. 2012;361:1–22. PubMed PMID: 22643916.

[23] Rhodes HM, Hirigoyen D, Shabnam L, Williams DN, Hansen GT. Infective endocarditis due to *Abiotrophia defectiva* and Granulicatella sp. complicated by infectious intracranial cerebral aneurysms: a report of 3 cases and review of the literature. J Med Microbiol. 2016 Apr 5 65(6):493–9. PubMed PMID: 27046228.

[24] Carleo MA, Del Giudice A, Viglietti R, Rosario P, Esposito V. Aortic valve endocarditis caused by *Abiotrophia defectiva*: case report and literature overview. In Vivo. 2015 Sep–Oct;29(5):515–8. PubMed PMID: 26359407.

[25] Brook I. Infective endocarditis caused by anaerobic bacteria. Arch Cardiovasc Dis. 2008 Oct;101(10):665–76. PubMed PMID: 19056073.

[26] Pachirat O, Watt G, Pussadhamma B. First case of tricuspid valve endocarditis caused by Gemella bergeri. Case Rep Med. 2015;2015:704785. PubMed PMID: 26294915. Pubmed Central PMCID: 4534595.

[27] Ramchandani MS, Rakita RM, Freeman RV, Levy WC, Von Homeyer P, Mokadam NA. Total artificial heart as bridge to transplantation for severe culture-negative prosthetic valve endocarditis due to Gemella haemolysans. ASAIO J. 2014 Jul–Aug;60(4):479–81. PubMed PMID: 24727539. Pubmed Central PMCID: 4375059.

[28] Gunes Y, Tuncer M, Guntekin U, Akdag S, Ali Gumrukcuoglu H, Karahocagil M, et al. Clinical characteristics and outcome of Brucella endocarditis. Trop Doct. 2009 Apr; 39(2):85–8. PubMed PMID: 19299289.

[29] Samuel V, Bajwa AA, Cury JD. First case of *Legionella pneumophila* native valve endocarditis. Int J Infect Dis. 2011 Aug;15(8):e576–7. PubMed PMID: 21641261.

[30] Thurneysen C, Boggian K. *Legionella pneumophila* serogroup 1 septic arthritis with probable endocarditis in an immunodeficient patient. J Clin Rheumatol. 2014 Aug; 20(5):297–8. PubMed PMID: 25057741.

[31] Bouchiat C, Saison J, Boisset S, Flandrois JP, Issartel B, Dauwalder O, et al. Nontuberculous mycobacteria: an underestimated cause of bioprosthetic valve infective endocarditis. Open forum infectious diseases. 2015 Apr;2(2):ofv047. PubMed PMID: 26213691. Pubmed Central PMCID: 4511745.

[32] Hooda A, Pati PK, John B, George PV, Michael JS. Disseminated *Mycobacterium chelonae* infection causing pacemaker lead endocarditis in an immunocompetent host. BMJ Case Reports. 2014;2014. PubMed PMID: 25535221.

[33] McMullen AR, Mattar C, Kirmani N, Burnham CA. Brown-pigmented Mycobacterium mageritense as a cause of prosthetic valve endocarditis and bloodstream infection. Journal of clinical microbiology. 2015 Aug;53(8):2777–80. PubMed PMID: 26063854. Pubmed Central PMCID: 4508415.

[34] Bartels H, Goldenberger D, Reuthebuch O, Vosbeck J, Weisser M, Frei R, et al. First case of infective endocarditis caused by *Helicobacter cinaedi*. BMC infectious diseases. 2014;14:586. PubMed PMID: 25403102. Pubmed Central PMCID: 4243372.

[35] Nishida K, Iwasawa T, Tamura A, Lefor AT. Infected abdominal aortic aneurysm with *Helicobacter cinaedi*. Case reports in surgery. 2016;2016:1396568. PubMed PMID: 26885430. Pubmed Central PMCID: 4739218.

[36] Siciliano RF, Castelli JB, Mansur AJ, Pereira dos Santos F, Colombo S, do Nascimento EM, et al. *Bartonella* spp. and *Coxiella burnetii* associated with community-acquired, culture-negative endocarditis, Brazil. Emerging Infectious Diseases. 2015 Aug;21(8): 1429–32. PubMed PMID: 26197233. Pubmed Central PMCID: 4517744.

[37] Keynan Y, MacKenzie L, Lagace-Wiens P. Quintessential culture-negative endocarditis. The Canadian Journal of Cardiology. 2016 Mar;32(3):395 e9–e10. PubMed PMID: 26342845.

[38] Edouard S, Nabet C, Lepidi H, Fournier PE, Raoult D. Bartonella, a common cause of endocarditis: a report on 106 cases and review. Journal of Clinical Microbiology. 2015 Mar;53(3):824–9. PubMed PMID: 25540398. Pubmed Central PMCID: 4390654.

[39] Georgievskaya Z, Nowalk AJ, Randhawa P, Picarsic J. *Bartonella henselae* endocarditis and glomerulonephritis with dominant C3 deposition in a 21-year-old male with a Melody transcatheter pulmonary valve: case report and review of the literature. Pediatric and Developmental Pathology: the Official Journal of the Society for Pediatric Pathology and the Paediatric Pathology Society. 2014 Jul–Aug;17(4):312–20. PubMed PMID: 24896298.

[40] Sosa T, Goldstein B, Cnota J, Bryant R, Frenck R, Washam M, et al. Melody valve *Bartonella henselae* endocarditis in an afebrile teen: a case report. Pediatrics. 2016 Jan; 137(1). PubMed PMID: 26659816.

[41] Sumatani I, Kagiyama N, Saito C, Makanae M, Kanetsuna H, Ahn K, et al. Infective endocarditis with negative blood culture and negative echocardiographic findings. Journal of Echocardiography. 2015 Jun;13(2):66–8. PubMed PMID: 26184640.

[42] Van Haare Heijmeijer S, Wilmes D, Aydin S, Clerckx C, Labriola L. Necrotizing ANCA-positive glomerulonephritis secondary to culture-negative endocarditis. Case Reports in Nephrology. 2015;2015:649763. PubMed PMID: 26819786. Pubmed Central PMCID: 4706874.

[43] Lemoine M, Edet S, Francois A, Bessin C, Guerrot D. Proliferative glomerulonephritis and erythroblastopenia associated with *Bartonella quintana* endocarditis [Glomerulonephrite proliferative et erythroblastopenie associees a une endocardite a *Bartonella quintana*]. Nephrologie & Therapeutique. 2015 Dec;11(7):569–72. PubMed PMID: 26404944.

[44] Verdier-Watts F, Peloni JM, Piegay F, Gerome P, Aussoleil A, Durand-de-Gevigney G, et al. An exceptional case of tricuspid infective endocarditis due to Bartonella henseale revealed by an old pulmonary embolism [Un cas exceptionnel d'endocardite infectieuse tricuspide a *Bartonella henselae* revelee par une embolie pulmonaire]. Annales de Cardiologie et d'angeiologie. 2016 Feb;65(1):48–50. PubMed PMID: 25869466.

[45] Raoult D, Tissot-Dupont H, Foucault C, Gouvernet J, Fournier PE, Bernit E, et al. Q fever 1985–1998. Clinical and epidemiologic features of 1,383 infections. Medicine. 2000 Mar;79(2):109–23. PubMed PMID: 10771709.

[46] Ngatchou W, Stefanidis C, Ramadan AS, De Canniere D. Recurrent endocarditis of a bicuspid aortic valve due to Q fever. Interactive cardiovascular and thoracic surgery. 2007 Dec;6(6):815–7. PubMed PMID: 17693439.

[47] Briggs BJ, Raoult D, Hijazi ZM, Edouard S, Angelakis E, Logan LK. Coxiella burnetii endocarditis in a child caused by a new genotype. The Pediatric Infectious Disease Journal. 2016 Feb;35(2):213–4. PubMed PMID: 26535879.

[48] Marth T, Moos V, Muller C, Biagi F, Schneider T. *Tropheryma whipplei* infection and Whipple's disease. The Lancet Infectious Diseases. 2016 Mar;16(3):e13–22. PubMed PMID: 26856775.

[49] Alozie A, Zimpfer A, Koller K, Westphal B, Obliers A, Erbersdobler A, et al. Arthralgia and blood culture-negative endocarditis in middle age men suggest *Tropheryma whipplei* infection: report of two cases and review of the literature. BMC Infectious Diseases. 2015;15:339. PubMed PMID: 26282628. Pubmed Central PMCID: 4539700.

[50] Gruber JR, Sarro R, Delaloye J, Surmely JF, Siniscalchi G, Tozzi P, et al. *Tropheryma whipplei* bivalvular endocarditis and polyarthralgia: a case report. Journal of Medical Case Reports. 2015;9:259. PubMed PMID: 26577283. Pubmed Central PMCID: 4650277.

[51] Herrmann MD, Neumayr A, Essig A, Spiess J, Merk J, Moller P, et al. Isolated Whipple's endocarditis: an underestimated diagnosis that requires molecular analysis of surgical material. The Annals of Thoracic Surgery. 2014 Jul;98(1):e1–3. PubMed PMID: 24996742.

[52] Thuny F, Fournier PE, Casalta JP, Gouriet F, Lepidi H, Riberi A, et al. Investigation of blood culture-negative early prosthetic valve endocarditis reveals high prevalence of fungi. Heart. 2010 May;96(10):743–7. PubMed PMID: 19910288.

[53] Kalokhe AS, Rouphael N, El Chami MF, Workowski KA, Ganesh G, Jacob JT. Aspergillus endocarditis: a review of the literature. International Journal of Infectious Diseases: IJID: Official Publication of the International Society for Infectious Diseases. 2010 Dec;14(12):e1040–7. PubMed PMID: 21036091.

[54] Kodali A, Khalighi K. A case of late implantable cardiac device infection with Aspergillus in an immunocompetent host. The American Journal of Case Reports. 2015;16:520–3. PubMed PMID: 26250569. Pubmed Central PMCID: 4530982.

[55] Rao U, O'Sullivan M. Lesson of the month (2). An unique presentation of infective endocarditis. Clinical Medicine. 2011 Dec;11(6):625–6. PubMed PMID: 22268325.

[56] Jinno S, Gripshover BM, Lemonovich TL, Anderson JM, Jacobs MR. *Histoplasma capsulatum* prosthetic valve endocarditis with negative fungal blood cultures and negative histoplasma antigen assay in an immunocompetent patient. Journal of Clinical Microbiology. 2010 Dec;48(12):4664–6. PubMed PMID: 20926709. Pubmed Central PMCID: 3008473.

[57] Ledtke C, Rehm SJ, Fraser TG, Shrestha NK, Tan CD, Rodriguez ER, et al. Endovascular infections caused by *Histoplasma capsulatum*: a case series and review of the literature. Archives of pathology & laboratory medicine. 2012 Jun;136(6):640–5. PubMed PMID: 22646271.

[58] Lorchirachonkul N, Foongladda S, Ruangchira-Urai R, Chayakulkeeree M. Prosthetic valve endocarditis caused by *Histoplasma capsulatum*: the first case report in Thailand.

Journal of the Medical Association of Thailand = Chotmaihet thangphaet. 2013 Feb;96 Suppl 2:S262–5. PubMed PMID: 23590052.

[59] Izumi K, Hisata Y, Hazama S. A rare case of infective endocarditis complicated by Trichosporon asahii fungemia treated by surgery. Annals of Thoracic and Cardiovascular Surgery: Official Journal of the Association of Thoracic and Cardiovascular Surgeons of Asia. 2009 Oct;15(5):350–3. PubMed PMID: 19901894.

[60] Rath PC, Purohit BV, Agrawal B, Reddy K, Nutankavala L, Narreddy S, et al. Pacemaker lead endocarditis due to Trichosporon species. The Journal of the Association of Physicians of India. 2015 Apr;63(4):66–8. PubMed PMID: 26591175.

[61] Badiee P, Amirghofran AA, Ghazi Nour M. Evaluation of noninvasive methods for the diagnosis of fungal endocarditis. Medical Mycology. 2014 Jul;52(5):530–6. PubMed PMID: 24915853.

[62] Tattevin P, Revest M, Lefort A, Michelet C, Lortholary O. Fungal endocarditis: current challenges. International Journal of Antimicrobial Agents. 2014 Oct;44(4):290–4. PubMed PMID: 25178919.

[63] Jos SL, Angelakis E, Caus T, Raoult D. Positron emission tomography in the diagnosis of Whipple's endocarditis: a case report. BMC Research Notes. 2015;8:56. PubMed PMID: 25889155. Pubmed Central PMCID: 4345011.

[64] Thadani SR, Dyverfeldt P, Gin A, Chitsaz S, Rao RK, Hope MD. Comprehensive evaluation of culture-negative endocarditis with use of cardiac and 4-dimensional-flow magnetic resonance imaging. Texas Heart Institute journal/from the Texas Heart Institute of St Luke's Episcopal Hospital, Texas Children's Hospital. 2014 Jun;41(3):351–2. PubMed PMID: 24955064. Pubmed Central PMCID: 4060342.

[65] Jordana-Lluch E, Gimenez M, Quesada MD, Rivaya B, Marco C, Dominguez MJ, et al. Evaluation of the broad-range PCR/ESI-MS technology in blood specimens for the molecular diagnosis of bloodstream infections. PloS One. 2015;10(10):e0140865. PubMed PMID: 26474394. Pubmed Central PMCID: 4608784.

[66] Inacio RC, Klautau GB, Murca MA, da Silva CB, Nigro S, Rivetti LA, et al. Microbial diagnosis of infection and colonization of cardiac implantable electronic devices by use of sonication. International Journal of Infectious Diseases: IJID: Official Publication of the International Society for Infectious Diseases. 2015 Sep;38:54–9. PubMed PMID: 26216762.

[67] Rohacek M, Erne P, Kobza R, Pfyffer GE, Frei R, Weisser M. Infection of cardiovascular implantable electronic devices: detection with sonication, swab cultures, and blood cultures. Pacing and clinical electrophysiology: PACE. 2015 Feb;38(2):247–53. PubMed PMID: 25377386.

[68] Fukui Y, Aoki K, Okuma S, Sato T, Ishii Y, Tateda K. Metagenomic analysis for detecting pathogens in culture-negative infective endocarditis. Journal of Infection and Chemo-

therapy: Official Journal of the Japan Society of Chemotherapy. 2015 Dec;21(12):882–4. PubMed PMID: 26360016.

[69] Haag H, Locher F, Nolte O. Molecular diagnosis of microbial aetiologies using SepsiTest in the daily routine of a diagnostic laboratory. Diagnostic Microbiology and Infectious Disease. 2013 Aug;76(4):413–8. PubMed PMID: 23747029.

[70] Brinkman CL, Vergidis P, Uhl JR, Pritt BS, Cockerill FR, Steckelberg JM, et al. PCR-electrospray ionization mass spectrometry for direct detection of pathogens and antimicrobial resistance from heart valves in patients with infective endocarditis. Journal of Clinical Microbiology. 2013 Jul;51(7):2040–6. PubMed PMID: 23596241. Pubmed Central PMCID: 3697732.

[71] Wallet F, Herwegh S, Decoene C, Courcol RJ. PCR-electrospray ionization time-of-flight mass spectrometry: a new tool for the diagnosis of infective endocarditis from heart valves. Diagnostic Microbiology and Infectious Disease. 2013 Jun;76(2):125–8. PubMed PMID: 23523601.

[72] Habib G, Lancellotti P, Antunes MJ, Bongiorni MG, Casalta JP, Del Zotti F, et al. 2015 ESC Guidelines for the management of infective endocarditis: The Task Force for the Management of Infective Endocarditis of the European Society of Cardiology (ESC). Endorsed by: European Association for Cardio-Thoracic Surgery (EACTS), the European Association of Nuclear Medicine (EANM). European Heart Journal. 2015 Nov 21;36(44):3075–128. PubMed PMID: 26320109.

[73] Tattevin P, Mainardi JL. Analysis of the 2015 American and European guidelines for the management of infective endocarditis. Med Mal Infect. 2016 Jun 10. pii: S0399-077X(16)30049-X. doi: 10.1016/j.medmal.2016.05.008. [Epub ahead of print] Review. PMID:27297743.

Section 4

Special Problems

Chapter 7

Infective Endocarditis in End-Stage Renal Disease Patients in Developing Countries: What is the Real Problem?

Díaz-García Héctor Rafael,
Contreras-de la Torre Nancy Anabel,
Alemán-Villalobos Alfonso,
Carrillo-Galindo María de Jesús,
Gómez-Jiménez Olivia Berenice,
Esparza-Beléndez Edgar,
Ramírez-Rosales Gladys Eloísa,
Portilla-d Buen Eliseo and Arreola-Torres Ramón

Additional information is available at the end of the chapter

http://dx.doi.org/10.5772/64929

Abstract

The epidemiology of infective endocarditis (IE) has changed over the last decades, due to various factors. This chapter focuses on IE in patients with end-stage renal disease. Then it reviews the most relevant reports published in the last decade worldwide; the different scenarios in developing countries versus developed countries; different microorganisms, treatment times, and outcomes; and also our own experience in these patients. Finally, it mentions the recommendations that have helped some developed countries to reduce more than 50% of bacteremia in catheter patients and how to make them possible in developing countries.

Keywords: end-stage renal disease (ESRD), developing countries, hemodialysis (HD), infective endocarditis (IE), catheter-related bacteremia (CRB), rheumatic heart disease (RHD)

1. Introduction

The epidemiology of infectious endocarditis (IE) has changed over the past five decades, with many contributing factors for the increasing incidence. The survival rate of chronically ill patients with nephropathy and cardiac patients has increased by transplanting or immunosuppressing, which is a consequence of medical advances. All risk factors in certain subgroups of patients are associated with the use of intracardiac or intravascular devices, prosthetic implants or catheters, and immunosuppressive drugs, causing increased health care-related infections. Despite advances in medicine, in-hospital mortality rate of IE remains high with no significant decrease observed since the 1960s [1].

Despite many scientific efforts that have been made to realize the magnitude of this problem in different regions of the world, assessing its incidence is difficult because of the few epidemiological studies that currently exist globally; the incidence of endocarditis may vary from one country to another, between 1.5 and 11.6 per 100,000 inhabitants. Apart from its incidence, it is recognizing that this is a condition that involves high morbidity and mortality [2].

Infective endocarditis (IE) in patients with end-stage renal disease (ESRD) is a problem that continues *in crescendo* worldwide, with high morbidity and mortality, but in developing countries, the problem is more alarming due to various factors such as underdevelopment, economic inequality, and limitations in health care systems. The treatment has not changed in recent decades and instead epidemiological characteristics show very specific changes that vary from the developed countries to developing countries [3, 4].

Some authors have proposed modifications in the IE classification to address hemodialysis (HD) patients in a different category, because they represent a crescent population of IE patients and diagnostic and treatment challenge for clinicians and surgeons [5].

This chapter highlights some identified differences as well as some regional differences between developed and developing countries, and provides strategies to reduce IE in HD patients, which can be performed in any health care facility.

2. Epidemiology

The precise incidence of IE is difficult to ascertain because case definition has varied over time between authors and clinical centers [6].

IE varies according to the region. Limited data suggest that the characteristics of IE in low-income countries differ from those in industrialized countries. It is estimated that over 33,700 rheumatic heart disease (RHD)-related IE cases arise each year in developing countries and that this leads to over 8400 deaths [7].

Many literature reports and a few retrospective series have been presented on infective endocarditis in the hemodialysis population. The true incidence of IE in HD patients is, at best, an underestimate in retrospective studies. It is reported that it occurs in 6% of HD patients.

http://dx.doi.org/10.5772/64929

The incidence of IE in HD patients is estimated to be 308/100,000 patient-years, which is 50- to 180-fold higher than 1.7–6.2 cases per 100,000 patient-years reported for the general population [8].

In a recent retrospective cohort study in Taiwan undertaken to determine IE and the mortality risk factors among HD patients, the prevalence of IE of 6.9% was reported. The overall mortality in HD patients with IE was 60.0% [9]. The mortality rate is also higher (30–77.8%) in HD patients than in IE patients in the general population (17%) [4]. There is a high postoperative mortality 11–80% in HD patients which requires surgical intervention for IE [10].

3. The ESRD patients in dialysis

The main risk factors for HD patients to get IE are recurrent bacteremia, uremia, immune-system damage, and premature degeneration of the heart valves caused by abnormalities in calcium and phosphorus homeostasis and chronic inflammation [8].

In 2006 the National Kidney Foundation established their guideline recommendations to select and place the access of HD being first choice arteriovenous fistula followed by fistula with synthetic graft leaving tunneled catheters and nontunneled as an alternative only when you do not have any of the first two options. Despite the goal since these guidelines were made in 2006 to have 50% of HD in AVF, this percentage has been achieved only in some European countries, but in North America, it has less percentage than what the guidelines suggest [11].

Mechanical and infectious complications most frequently limit the use of a central venous catheter (CVC). Infection is the most common cause of morbidity and the second cause of death after cardiovascular disease in HD patients. The incidence of catheter-related bacteremia (CRB) in HD patients depends on the type and location of the CVC, the characteristics of the population, insertion techniques and safety measures, and manipulation of HD catheters in each center. The CRB rate in nontunneled CVC is between 3.8 and 6.6 episodes/1000 days of the use of CVC and between 1.6 and 5.5 episodes/1000 days of the use of tunneled CVC. The use of a tunneled CVC carries an increased risk of bacteremia 7 to 20 times compared to the arteriovenous fistulas (AVF) [12].

The International Collaboration on Endocarditis Prospective Cohort Study conducted a prospective cohort study with 2781 adults diagnosed with infective endocarditis in 58 hospitals in 25 countries from June 2000 to September 2005, which reported an IE incidence of 21% in chronic HD patients (more than 90 days) and 25% chronic IV access in North America; 8% in chronic HD patients and 5% chronic IV access in South America; and 4% in chronic HD patients and 5% chronic IV access in Europe [13].

The above statistics differ from those reported by other authors from different parts of the world; UK presents a lower incidence of reported cases of endocarditis; and Doulton Timothy et al. reported a series of 28 cases of IE using the Duke criteria, at St. Thomas' Hospital (1980–1995), Guy's (1995–2002), and King's College Hospitals (1996–2002). Of this

28 patients, 27 patients were on chronic HD and 1 in peritoneal dialysis (PD) patient. 40% of the HD patients were treated with AVF's and the AVF was the definite or suspected site of entry for the causative organism in eight cases of IE representing the 26.6% of the total of patients with IE. The presumption that the AVF was the source of bacteremia in these episodes is supported by the fact that the causative organism in seven episodes was commensal skin pathogens *Staphylococcus aureus* (*S. aureus*) in six patients and *Staphylococcus epidermidis* (*S. epidermidis*) in one patient [3]. In contrast, Jones et al. conducted a retrospective study between the years 1998 and 2011. Forty-two patients were identified with developed IE out of a total incident dialysis population of 1500 over 13 years. Ninety-five percent of patients (40/42) were on long-term HD and five percent (2/42) on PD. Mean patient age was 55.2 years (IQR: 43–69), and the mean duration of HD prior to IE was 57.4 months. Primary HD access at the time of diagnosis was an AVF in 35% (14/40), a dual-lumen tunneled catheter (DLTC) in 55% (22/40), and a dual-lumen nontunneled catheter (DLNTC) in 10% (4/40). *S. aureus*, including methicillin-resistant *S. aureus* (MRSA), was present in 57.1% (24/42) [14, 15].

4. IE risk factors in dialysis patients

Dialysis is a well-established risk factor for IE. Mylonakis et al. reported that end-stage renal disease in HD patients has a higher rate of morbidity and mortality compared to general population. Infections are the major cause of morbidity and mortality and are the second leading cause of death in HD patients surpassed only by cardiovascular disease. And these occur in about 12–22% of ESRD patients [15–17].

The mortality rate in patients with IE ranges from 30 to 56% in one year and in-hospital mortality is twice more frequent than the general population with IE.

4.1. HD-related bacteremia

One of the factors that increase the risk of developing IE in HD patients is bacteremia, which are exposed to repetitive vascular access through an arteriovenous fistula (AVF), polytetrafluoroethylene (PTFE) grafts or percutaneous catheters for HD, or cuffed or noncuffed dual lumen catheter.

The incidence of bacteremia is related to vascular access type, ranging from 1.6 to 7.7 per 1000 days with percutaneous catheters and 0.2 to 0.5 per 1000 days with AVF, according to the reference.

The use of catheters during HD is the leading cause of bacteremia in HD patients [4, 8, 15, 18].

A hierarchy of bacteremia risk exists among various types of HD vascular access; it is less common in patients with native arteriovenous fistulae, while synthetic grafts, cuffed catheters, and uncuffed catheters yield a progressively increasing risk.

These episodes of bacteremia during HD are relatively common. They can be endogenous or exogenous: through the microorganism flora found in the patient (endogenous) or through

http://dx.doi.org/10.5772/64929

the pathogen from another source such as might occur through hands or contaminated instruments (exogenous) [5].

There are three points where the pathogens can enter the bloodstream (BS):

(a) Product contamination of the infusion.

Contamination of parenteral fluids is exceptional at the present time due to the rigorous control sterility and subject to quick degradation once the expiration date is reached. In these cases, bacteremia usually caused by Gram-negative bacteria (Enterobacteriaceae or nonfermenting Gram-negative bacilli) particularly serious and epidemic type may occur.

(b) Contamination of connection and intraluminal space.

Contamination of the connection point of vascular catheters is the second most common cause of arrival of microorganisms to the bloodstream (after related to the place of insertion) and the most common involved in intravascular devices longer than 2 weeks. It is, therefore, the usual way of colonization of CVC, whether or not tunneled, when it occurs after 2 weeks from implantation. In this way, microorganism colonizations progress through the intraluminal surface of catheters, forming biofilm colonization all the way from the outside end to the intravascular end.

(c) Contamination adjacent to the site of insertion and extraluminal surface skin.

Access to microorganisms from the skin adjacent the insertion site of the catheter is the most common for colonization and subsequent infection-related pathogenic mechanism. This is the only way for a microorganism to get into the bloodstream in the first 8 days (in the absence of product contamination infusion). Microorganisms on the skin through the insertion point enter the extraluminal surface of catheters and form the biofilm at that level to the intravascular end.

Another option of extraluminal contamination of a vascular catheter colonization can be by hematogenous spread of a microorganism originated in a distant focus, which is very rare, observed mainly in critically ill patients with long-term catheters or in patients with intestinal diseases [19].

4.2. Degenerative heart valve disease (DHVD)

Patients with ESRD have increased incidence of degenerative disease of the heart valves, which is one of the major risks of IE. The calcific aortic stenosis and mitral annular calcification with consequent failure are the most common diseases. It has been found that this condition occurs prematurely in this group of patients 10–20 years prior to the general population. Degenerative heart valve disease is caused due to disorders of calcium and phosphorus homeostasis, in the setting of secondary hyperparathyroidism, and due to the chronic micro-inflammatory milieu of uremia associated with ESRD [5].

4.3. Rheumatic heart disease (RHD)

The RHD, which was the leading cause of IE in the preantibiotics era, is now rare in developed countries. However, it remains a highly prevalent disease in developing countries. More developed areas, such as Hong Kong and Thailand, still have a case of IE in 18 and 12%, respectively.

Chou et al. in their study compared 68,426 adult patients with ESRD in HD with two groups: with IE and without IE. They found that 1.2% without IE and 4.4% with IE, respectively, had the RHD, having a statistical significance $p < 0.001$, relative to RHD and IE in HD patients [16]. The same study shows the differences in incidence among Asian countries and the western countries. However, many western countries, such as in the case of Mexico and parts of South America, are still considered to be endemic for this disease. Simsek-Yavuz et al. in their study in Turkey also noted the difference in incidence among the developed countries and found low incidence of RHD compared with developing countries. They presented their work in 325 patients with IE that 33% had RHD.

Although this study is not specifically for HD patients, it demonstrates a high prevalence of RHD in IE [20].

4.4. Chronic degenerative diseases (CDD)

- *Diabetes*

There is a close relationship between HD patients and diabetes, with the incidence of IE.

There are studies that have an incidence of 33–59.4% of patients having statistical significance compared with HD patients with DM without IE, $p < 0.001$ [15, 16].

- *Systemic hypertension*

This condition is related to ESRD patients with HD and IE having an incidence of up 89.9% [15].

- *Coronary artery disease (CAD)*

Kamalakannan et al. in their study with 69 patients showed an incidence of 24.6% of CAD in HD patients with IE. Chou et al. found $p < 0.001$ between HD patients with IE versus the HD patient without IE. This disease is considered to be a potential cause of death in the short and long term in these patients [8, 15, 16].

- *Congestive heart failure (CHF)*

Kamalakannan et al. in their study with 69 patients showed an incidence of 18.8% of CHF in this group of patients. Chou et al. compared CHF in HD patients with IE versus HD patients without IE and found significant differences $p < 0.001$, being the HD patients with IE, the group with more CHF, which also indicates the direct cause of death in these patients in the short term [8, 15, 16].

4.5. Preexisiting cardiac abnormalities

These account for 13.5–33.3% of the causes associated with IE in HD patients, and include the presence of valve prostheses, previous valvular heart disease, heart transplantation, pericarditis, myocarditis, and intracardiac devices.

The incidence of cardiac device infective endocarditis (CDIE) has been reported between 0.06 and 0.6% per year or 1.14 per 1000 device-years [15, 16, 21].

4.6. Intravenous drug users

Although it is a rare case of IE in HD patients, Kamalakannan et al. reported an incidence of 11.6% representing eight patients of the study [8]. Also in some countries such as Finland they found an increase in IV drug abuse as a risk factor for IE patients being 0% in the 1980s and mid-1990s to 20% in 2000–2004 [22].

4.7. Elderly patients

A relationship has been found between the advanced ages of the patient with ESRD on HD; some authors considered ≥ 65 years and others ≥ 70 years with IE. Nori et al. reported a frequency of IE 27%, the highest among age groups for patients ≥ 70 years. Chou et al. reported 48% of HD patients with IE ≥ 65 years. The ages of the Patients in HD with IE were 62.12 ± 13.09 years versus 60.11 ± 14.06 years in HD patients without IE, resulting in a $p < 0.001$, confirming that the advanced age is a risk factor for IE. Watt et al. presented a comparison of patients treated in Rennes, France, versus patients treated in Khon Kaen, Thailand (from rural areas in Thailand), finding a statistical difference in the age with an average of 70 versus 47 years, respectively.

Also elderly patients are considered to have a poor prognostic factor in IE in HD patients.

Also older age is a determinant of the clinical features in IE. Fewer patients can go to surgical treatment and mortality is higher than in younger patients [7, 13, 15, 16, 23].

4.8. Methicillin-susceptible *Staphylococcus aureus* (MSSA) and methicillin-resistant *Staphylococcus aureus* (MRSA) infection

Staphylococcus aureus represents the primary pathogen in IE in HD patients causing up to 80% of the IE. This pathogen is much more frequent than in the general population with IE. This can be explained that more than 50% of patients in dialysis are carriers of *S. aureus*; nose as a reservoir has shown an increased risk of subsequent infections. It is also important to consider that this pathogen by the fact is responsible for a high number of septic complications compared with other microorganisms. Finally, recent studies have shown that as much as 50% of *S. aureus* IE is MRSA. These strains in particular are more difficult to eradicate and are associated with a worse prognosis than methicillin-susceptible *S. aureus*. In general, patients with MRSA got it as an in-hospital infection; however, studies have shown the existence of community-acquired strains, which are microbiologically different from those acquired during hospitalization. Those strains are called community-acquired *Staphylococcus aureus* methicillin-resistant (CA-MRSA). It is a predisposing factor in these patients and a challenge for physicians involved with patients with MRSA IE [1, 5, 24].

4.9. Other microorganisms

Streptococcus viridans is currently considered to be the second cause of IE after *S. aureus*. Other pathogens such as *Enterococci* occupy the third place. The relevance of the latter is that its incidence has been increasing, plus it is more associated with nosocomial infection compared with *Streptococcus*. These pathogens if presented in prosthetic valves are more likely to cause intracardiac abscesses and less likely to have detectable vegetations on echocardiography than those presented in IE in native valves [1].

4.10. Immunosuppression

In patients with ESRD, there is a malfunction in polymorphonuclear and mobility of granulocytes, which reduce defense of the patient's cells, thus failing to remove bacteria from the bloodstream properly [5].

5. Heart valves with IE in HD

As mentioned earlier the incidence of IE in HD patients is higher than in general population and it is caused by multiple factors. But it is closely related to frequent episodes of bacteremia related to dialysis access and the predisposition of these patients to present premature degeneration of the heart valves eventually causing bacterial implantation in the valves. This is an issue of major public health presenting a very poor prognosis in short and long term, with 23.5% in-hospital mortality and 61.6% mortality in 1 year.

Despite the high rates of IE and poor prognosis for these patients, there has not been a substantial change in mortality over the past two decades. This can be the result of not having important changes in the therapeutic armamentarium [25]. Reports of multiple studies have shown that left valves with IE in HD patients are affected twice the time compared to the right valves; as well as the mitral valve is affected in more patients than the aortic valve. It is theorized that the thickening of these valves, which is common in this group of patients, can lead to increased susceptibility to acquire IE because of alterations in the laminar flow. Mitral annular calcification, which is also common in ESRD, has also shown increased susceptibility to IE [8].

5.1. Transthoracic echocardiogram (TTE) versus transesophageal echocardiogram (TEE)

TTE as a first-line diagnostic tool can work, but Kamalakannan et al. reported only 55.3% positive for vegetations in IE in HD and after using TEE 92.5% were positive for vegetations [8].

5.2. Medical treatment

Medical treatment for IE in HD patients, if considering the current guidelines for IE in general population, must have some important considerations in this group of patients.

Vancomycin should not be used in IE with MSSA, because of two reasons: (1) its low bactericidal activity when compared with oxacillin or cefazolin and (2) its main role in strains of *S. aureus* with reduced glycopeptides and vancomycin-resistant *Enterococci* sensitivity. Conversely, when dealing with a patient with IE with MRSA, vancomycin (possibly in combination with rifampicin) remains the drug of choice, if it is possible to obtain and maintain plasma levels between 15 and 20 mg/L without toxicity [5].

5.3. Surgical treatment

You can repair a valve anytime with a TEE confirmation of good valve function, which is better than replacement.

Valve replacement is a key part of therapy in patients with IE [25]. A large retrospective study by Rankin et al. used the Society of Thoracic Surgeons national database to analyze 1862 valve surgery operations in dialysis patients with endocarditis from 1994 to 2003 and reported an operative mortality of 24.4%. In this study, several risk factors for hospital mortality were proposed in HD patients with IE, including (salvage surgery/shock, surgery on both valves, elderly, affected mitral valve, high BMI, arrhythmias, active endocarditis, and female gender) [26]. A more recent study of Leither et al. found lower mortality in patients who underwent surgery of left-sided surgery compared to those reported by Ranki et al.

Current indications for surgery in a patient with IE (general population) according to the guidelines are valve disease causing CHF, recurrent emboli, persistent despite appropriate antibiotic treatment infection, and mobile and large vegetation formation of myocardial abscesses. However, these recommendations are made for IE general population; currently, there are no specific guidelines for IE in HD patients, taking into account that this indication may be debatable for these patients. Dialysis patients have a higher risk for mortality in the context of IE, lower life expectancy, high surgical risk, and often other associated morbidities [25]. In this context, there are some studies with very different results: Spies et al. reported 73% mortality and Kamalakannan et al. reported 80% survival in patients undergoing surgery, in in-hospital survival and only 43% survival with medical treatment. However, in the study of Kamalakannan et al. 12 of the 15 patients (80%) survived, but 24 of the 69 patients had indication for surgery according to the guidelines of IE for the general population, indicating that selection bias likely strongly influenced the outcomes reported in these studies [8, 25, 27].

About surgical treatment in this group of patients, there has always been controversy over what type of prosthesis to be used: biological or mechanical. These controversies started from two studies from the 1970s that were case series ($n = 4$ patients) in dialysis, where accelerated calcification of biological valves was documented. Now there are enough studies that compare the use of mechanical versus. bioprosthesis with no significant differences. Thourani et al., in 2011, demonstrated a in HD patients with IE patients undergoing valve replacement of 18.1%, with no difference between mechanical and bioprosthetic after 10 years [28]. Other studies have shown a higher incidence of bleeding and cerebrovascular events in patients with mechanical valves compared with bioprosthesis. In addition to oral anticoagulants, which are problematic in ESRD patients, most patients are prone to bleeding.

Since no significant differences are found between the types of valve prosthesis to be placed in HD patients with IE, it is recommended to individualize each case. But as a general rule, bioprosthesis is placed in most HD patients with IE, especially in patients with increased risk of bleeding associated with anticoagulation, leaving mechanical prostheses for young patients without other morbidity in whom life expectancy is longer than the bioprosthesis and also, for young patients who are candidates for renal transplantation in the future [25].

6. IE in HD patients in western Mexico

Our group works at a reference center, in the Mexican Institute of Social Security (IMSS for its acronym in Spanish) and takes care of all cardiothoracic surgical patients in the west of Mexico that are affiliated to IMSS. This means that more than 10 states represent more than 8.5 million affiliated people and possible patients. There are other hospitals in western Mexico that deal with endocarditis patients, but a patient who has surgical indication or who is seriously ill is sent to our center.

We retrospectively analyzed the last 5 year cases of IE in our center. There were 173 cases of which 77 (44.5%) were surgically treated. In these 77 patients, 33 (42.85%) patient where in HD. We used the IE in general population guidelines for the decision of medical or surgical treatment in all our patients.

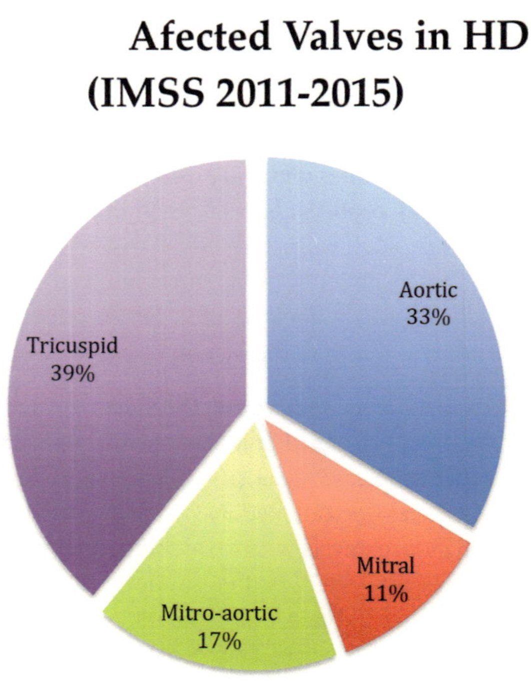

Figure 1. Affected valves in HD patients (IMSS 2011–2015).

In contrast to what previous publications have described regarding IE in HD patients, the most commonly infected valve in our surgical population was the tricuspid valve (**Figure 1**). Also, having a mean age of 38.5 years ranging between 19 and 76 years, which is significantly lower than previous reports. We consider that this can be related to the long mean time of nontunneled HD catheters observed in our patients and also for not having proper safety protocols for the prevention of bacteremia in the HD facilities. This also could be caused by Mexico's overpopulation in public health services and the long-lasting waiting list for AVFs or kidney transplantation, causing good transplant candidates to end up as chronic dialysis patients and making them more susceptible to bacteremia and infections. Even though our hospital is the leading center for kidney transplantation in all Latin America, the waiting list is affected by the overpopulation commented before.

7. Differences between case series of IE in ESRD patients

The following tables summarizes some of the most representative contemporary case series of IE in ESRD patients published in the last decade. The percentage of HD patients with IE who are undergoing cardiac surgery ranges from 7.8 to 53% in different regions of the world and also the associated pathologies are listed in **Table 1**. *S. aureus* is the microorganism most frequently involved in all series (**Table 1**). The valves involve with IE in previous studies involved most frequently the left side valves (**Table 2**). There are significant differences in the percentage of ESRD patients with AVFs in different regions, the highest being in Europe (**Table 3**). And morbidity and mortality also differ between regions (**Table 4**).

Authors	**Doulton T, Sabharwal N, Cairns H, *et al.***	**Jones D, McGill L, Rathod K, *et al.***	**Nori U, Manoharan A, Thornby J, *et al.***	**Kamalakannan D, Manohara R, Johnson L, et al.**	**Chou M, Wang J, Wu W, et al.**	**Chang C, Kuc B, Chen T, et al.**	**Baroudi S, Qazi R, Lentine K, et al.**
Journal	**Kidney International, 2003; 64: 720-727**	**Nephron Clinical Practice, 2013; 123: 151–156**	**Nephrology Dialysis Transplantation 2006; 21: 2184–2190**	**Annals of Thoracic Surgery 2007; 83: 2081–2086**	**Inter national Journal of Cardiology 2015; 179: 465–469**	**Journal of Nephro logy 2004; 17:228-235**	**NDT PLUS Nephrology Dialysis Transplantation**
Year	**2003**	**2013**	**2006**	**2007**	**2015**	**2004**	**2008**
Country	UK	UK	USA	USA	Taiwan	Taiwan	USA
Years of the study	**22**	**13**	**5**	**15**	**9**	**15**	**16**

Years in which the study was conducted	1980–1995, 1995–2002, 1996–2002	1998–2011	1999–2004	1990–2004	1999–2007	1988–2002	1990–2006
Participant centers	St. Thomas H. Guy´s H. King´s College H. (London)	Royal London Hospital. (London)	Columbus, Ohio Detroit, Michigan Houston, Texas	St. John Hospital and Medical Center. Detroit, Michigan.	National	Taipei Veterans General Hospital.	Saint Louis University Hospital.
IE patients (n)	28 pts.	42 pts.	52 pts.	69 pts.	502 (39 surgical)-7.8	20 pts.	59 pts.
Cardiac surgery	53% (15/28 pts.)	21% (9/42 pts.)	24% (13/52 pts.)	34% (24/69 pts.)	7.8% (39 pts.)	*(20 /20 pts.)	12% (7/59 pts.)
Male patients	60.7% (17 pts.)	52.2% (22 pts.)	52%	45% (31 pts.)	35.9% (14 pts.)	(13 pts.)	47% (28 pts.)
Mean age	54.1 (22-81)	55.2 (43-69)	60 (36-82)	56 +-13	52.6 +- 11.7	64.6+-12.9	57.3 +- 13.8
Diabetic%	8	33.3% (14 pts.)	42% (22 pts.)	37.7% (26 pts.)	46.2% (18 pts.)	45% (9 pts.)	59% (35)
Hypertension %	*	66.6% (28 pts.)	79% (41 pts.)	89.9% (62 pts.)	NR	75% (15 pts.)	93% (55)
Immuno suppression %	*	9.5% (4 pts.)	*	(3 pts.)	NR	*	5% (3 pts.)
Staphylococcus aureus	63.3% MRSA	57.1% (24/42 pts.)	20% (11 pts.)	*	*	*	45% (27 pts.)

* For the type of stratification of patients in the publication, the data are present but not reported in this table. NR: not reported.

Table 1. Infective endocarditis publications in ESRD patients in dialysis surgical treatment: demographic information.

Authors	Doulton T, Sabharwal N, Cairns H, *et al.*	Jones D, McGill L, Rathod K, *et al.*	Nori U, Manoharan A, Thornby J, *et al.*	Kamalakannan D, Manohara R, Johnson L, et al.	Chou M, Wang J, Wu W, et al.	Chang C, Kuo B, Chen T, et al.	Baroudi S, Qazi R, Lentine K, et al.
Journal	Kidney International, 2003; 64: 720-727	Nephron Clinical Practice, 2013; 123:151–156	Nephrology Dialysis Transplantation 2006; 21: 2184–2190	Annals of Thoracic Surgery 2007; 83: 2081–2086	International Journal of Cardiology 2015; 179:465–469	Journal of Nephrology 2004; 17: 228–235	NDT PLUS Nephrology Dialysis Transplantation

Year	**2003**	**2013**	**2006**	**2007**	**2015**	**2004**	**2008**
Country	UK	UK	USA	USA	Taiwan	Taiwan	USA
Involved heart valve%							
Mitral	41.4%	30.9% (13/42 pts.)	50% (27 pts.)	*	*	64%	63% (37 pts.)
Aortic	37.9%	42.8% (18/42 pts.)	43% (23 pts.)	*	*	18%	17% (10 pts.)
Tricuspid	NR	5 pts.	19% (10 pts.)	*	*	9%	*
Mitral and aortic	17.2%	9.5% (4/42 pts.)	*	*	*	9%	*
Previous valve lesions	13 pts. (51.7%)	33.3% (14 pts.)	*	10.1% (7 pts.)	*	*	*
Previous valvular prosthesis	2 pts	9.5% (4 pts.)	13% (7 pts.)	4.3% (3 pts.)	*	*	*

* For the type of stratification of patients in the publication, the data are present but not reported in this table. NR: not reported.

Table 2. Infective endocarditis publications in ESRD patients in dialysis surgical treatment: involved heart valves.

Authors	**Doulton T, Sabharwal N, Cairns H, et al.**	**Jones D, McGill L, Rathod K, *et al.***	**Nori U, Manoharan A, Thornby J, *et al.***	**Kamalakannan D, Manohara R, Johnson L, et al.**	**Chou M, Wang J, Wu W, et al.**	**Chang C, Kuo B, Chen T, et al.**	**Baroudi S, Qazi R, Lentine K, et al.**
Journal	**Kidney International, 2003; 64: 720–727**	**Nephron Clinical Practice, 2013; 123:151–156**	**Nephrology Dialysis Transplantation 2006; 21: 2184–2190**	**Annals of Thoracic Surgery 2007; 83: 2081–2086**	**International Journal of Cardiology 2015; 179: 465–469**	**Journal of Nephrology 2004; 17: 228–235**	**NDT PLUS Nephrology Dialysis Transplantation**
Year	2003	2013	2006	2007	2015	2004	2008
Country	UK	UK	USA	USA	Taiwan	Taiwan	USA
Dialysis access route%							
PTFE graft	10.8%	NR	13% (7 pts.)	21.7% (15 pts.)	*	15% (3 pts.)	44.1% (26 pts.)
AVF	41.3%	35% (14/40 pts.)	4% (2 pts.)	11.6% (8 pts.)	*	25% (5 pts.)	5.1% (3 pts.)
Tunneled catheter DL	37.9%	55% (22/40 pts.)	72% (39 pts.)	66.7% (46 pts.)	*	5% (1 pt.)	26 pts.

Nontunneled catheter	3.4%	10% (4/40 pts.)	2% (1 pt.)	0 (0%)	*	55% (11 pts.)	2 pts.
Peritoneal dialysis	3.4% (1)	5% (2/42 pts.)	NR	0 (0%)	*		
Mean time of HD before IE	46.3 (1.5-180)	57.4 (9.7 -85.5)	*	37+-32	*	12.9+-19.1	52.9 +- 58

* For the type of stratification of patients in the publication, the data are present but not reported in this table. NR: not reported.

Table 3. Infective endocarditis publications in ESRD patients in dialysis surgical treatment: dialysis access route.

Authors	**Doulton T, Sabharwal N, Cairns H,** ***et al.***	**Jones D, McGill L, Rathod K,** ***et al.***	**Nori U, Manoharan A, Thornby J,** ***et al.***	**Kamalakannan D, Manohara R, Johnson L, et al.**	**Chou M, Wang J, Wu W, et al.**	**Chang C, Kuo B, Chen T, et al.**	**Baroudi S, Qazi R, Lentine K, et al.**
Journal	**Kidney International, 2003; 64: 720–727**	**Nephron Clinical Practice, 2013; 123:151–156**	**Nephrology Dialysis Transplantation 2006; 21: 2184–2190**	**Annals of Thoracic Surgery 2007; 83: 2081–2086**	**International Journal of Cardiology 2015; 179: 465–469**	**Journal of Nephrology 2004; 17: 228–235**	**NDT PLUS Nephrology Dialysis Transplantation**
Year	**2003**	**2013**	**2006**	**2007**	**2015**	**2004**	**2008**
Country	UK	UK	USA	USA	Taiwan	Taiwan	USA
Survival to discharge after surgery	14 pts (93.3%)	88.8% (8 pts.)	*	*	*	*	*
Survival 3 months after surgery	*	86.9%	*	*	66.5%	*	*
Survival 1 year after surgery	*	77%	*	*	58.4%	*	*
In-hospital mortality% nonsurgical patients	*	14.3%	19 pts. (37%).	*	23.5%	*	*
In-hospital mortality% surgical patients	1 pt. (6.9%)	11.1%	*	*	25.9%	*	*
Subsequent mortality	>50% 1 year survival	29.2% - 1 month	32.7% - 3 months	13 pts. Follow-up	*	*	*

* For the type of stratification of patients in the publication, the data are present but not reported in this table. NR: not reported.

Table 4. Infective endocarditis publications in ESRD patients in dialysis surgical treatment: survival, in-hospital mortality, and overall mortality.

http://dx.doi.org/10.5772/64929

8. Prevention and future considerations

After analyzing the literature of IE in different regions of the world, we found different pathogens depending on the endemic regions for some pathologies, for example, RHD, usage of antibiotic treatment before having a diagnosis, endemic zones for rare pathogens such as *Brucella* spp. in Turkey or even zoonosis reported by Watt et al. [7, 16, 20].

One of the recommendations for developing countries must be an adequate treatment and follow-up for group A beta-hemolytic streptococcus to prevent rheumatic fever and its cardiac complications, which is one of the most common causes of IE in general population and in HD 19 patients in developing countries [16].

There are many different scenarios between developed and developing countries, but we think that the security measures for prevention of bacteremia in HD can be achieved in any health care unit using HD program regardless of the place. Reducing bacteremia in HD patients will reduce their incidence of IE [16].

Pronovost et al. in their study made in 103 UCIs in Michigan used basic changes in their practice of catheter implantation and management. An evidence-based intervention resulted in a large and sustained reduction (up to 66%) in rates of catheter-related bloodstream infection that was maintained throughout the 18-month study period [29].

8.1. Michigan and bacteremia zero recommendations

1. Wash your hands

Wash your hands before inserting a central venous catheter (CVC). Bottom Line: Proper hand hygiene is required before and after palpating catheter insertion sites, as well as before and after inserting, replacing, accessing, repairing, or dressing an intravascular catheter. In addition, the use of gloves does not obviate the need for hand hygiene. Category IA: Proper hand hygiene procedures can be achieved through the use of either a waterless, alcohol-based product or an antibacterial soap and water with adequate rinsing.

2. Clean the skin with chlorhexidine

Bottom Line: Disinfect clean skin with an appropriate antiseptic before catheter insertion and during dressing changes. A 2% chlorhexidine-based preparation is the preferred solution, Category IA [29].

Chaiyakunapruk et al., in their meta-analysis compared chlorhexidine versus povidone-iodine solution for vascular catheter site care, finding that the use of chlorhexidine reduces the risk for catheter-related bloodstream infection by 49% [30]. The same authors in another study, published one year later, concluded that the use of chlorhexidine, rather than povidone, for central catheter site care resulted in a 1.6% decrease in the incidence of catheter-related bloodstream infection, a 0.23% decrease in the incidence of death, and savings of $113 per catheter used [31].

3. Use of full-barrier precautions during CVC insertion

Bottom Line: Maintain aseptic technique for the insertion of intravascular catheters. Category IA: Maximal sterile barrier precautions (e.g., cap, mask, sterile gown, sterile gloves, and large sterile drape) during the insertion of CVCs substantially reduce the incidence of catheter-related bloodstream infection (CR-BSI) compared with standard precautions (e.g., sterile gloves and small drapes) [29].

4. Avoid the femoral site

Bottom Line: A subclavian site is preferred for infection control purposes, although other factors (e.g., the potential for noninfectious and catheter-operator skill) should be considered for deciding where to place the catheter. Category IA: The site at which a catheter is placed influences the subsequent risk for catheter-related infection and phlebitis. For adults, lower extremity insertion sites are associated with a higher risk of infection than upper extremity sites. As a result, authorities recommend that CVCs be placed in the subclavian site instead of a jugular or femoral site to reduce the risk for infection [29].

5. Remove unnecessary central venous catheters

Bottom Line: Promptly remove any intravascular catheter that is no longer essential. Category IA: One of the most effective strategies for preventing CR-BSIs is to eliminate, or at least reduce, exposure to central venous catheters. The decision regarding the need for a catheter, however, is complex and therefore difficult to standardize into a practice guideline. Nonetheless, to reduce exposure to central venous catheters, the ICU team should adopt a strategy to systematically evaluate daily whether any catheters or tubes can be removed [29].

6. Hygienic management of catheters

Minimize the manipulation of the connections and clean the injection sites of the catheter with isopropyl alcohol 70° before its use. Category IA: Another characteristic of this study was that the people in charge of the catheters needed to do an auto-test online, assist to safety meetings before they can be part of the study [32]. This study was performed in 68% of all ICUs in Spain, with a reduction of 50% in the bacteremia related to catheter in a two-year period [19].

In addition to the intervention to reduce the rate of catheter-related bloodstream infection, the ICUs implemented the use of a daily goal to improve clinician-to-clinician communication within the ICU, an intervention to reduce the incidence of ventilator-associated pneumonia, and a comprehensive unit-based safety program to improve the safety culture. The period necessary for the implementation of each intervention was estimated to be 3 months [29].

8.2. Our recommendations for developing countries

After analyzing the literature and the results in the different countries and our own experience, we made some recommendations that could help any HD program in developing countries for reducing their bacteremia incidence, and thus reducing the risk of IE.

http://dx.doi.org/10.5772/64929

1. Form a HD team

They should be the only people involved in the HD process. This can be achieved by online auto-test of the use of catheters and the safety recommendations for it. This team must have a leader, who has to be in constant training through conferences and workshops. This must be transmitted to the whole group, also by training and evaluations. Having a checklist for every procedure could also help reduce errors or omissions in the process. The personnel involved in this HD team must be able to teach all the safety measures for the patient and their family members to avoid infection of any HD access. They must provide standardized knowledge about topics such as vascular access care, hand hygiene, risks related to catheter use, recognizing signs of infection, and instructions for access management when away from the dialysis unit.

2. Cardiac screening for all ESRD patients

An ESRD patient who is going to start HD treatment should have a cardiac screening to rule out previous cardiac pathology. A patient with a heart disease should be considered for closer monitoring.

3. Respect hierarchy in vascular access for HD

Before HD, always consider that the hierarchy of bacteremia risk exists among various types of HD vascular access; it is less common in patients with native arteriovenous fistulae, while synthetic grafts, cuffed catheters, and uncuffed catheters yield a progressively increasing risk.

4. Respect hierarchy in vascular access when using catheters for HD

In the case of using catheters, the hierarchy of bacteremia risk is less common in subclavian catheters, jugular catheters, and femoral catheters, progressively increasing risk.

5. Use the Michigan and bacteremia zero recommendations when using catheters

When using a catheter for HD, always take the six recommendations given above from Pronovost et al. made in ICUs in Michigan and Bacteremia Zero from Spain, which reduce more than 50% of catheter-related bacteremia.

6. Nasal cultures for all ESRD patients

Nasal cultures for *S. aureus* for new patients and serial cultures for chronic patients and use of nasal mupirocin are recommended.

7. Inspect and clean catheter exit sites

Exit sites should be routinely inspected for infection at every dialysis session, and subjected to swabbing and bacterial culture whenever infection is suspected.

8. Suspicion of IE in HD patients? Always use TEE

TTE if not conclusive TEE to rule out or confirm the diagnosis; if TTE conclusive, use TEE to rule out other cardiac lesions or unidentified vegetations in other valves.

9. Vancomycin not as prophylactic

Confirm IE in HD patients; do not use prophylactic vancomycin if you suspect any pathogen different from MRSA.

10. Mechanical prosthesis not the only option for IE in HD patients

Biological prosthesis is a good option for these patients; the heart team must individualize each case; and consider the benefits or disadvantages of mechanical or biological prosthesis.

9. Conclusion

Here we have addressed the different protocols and outcomes among developed countries due to ESRD patients' population, economy and health care differences in each country. This means that the recommendations of different associations and foundations have not been completely followed up by all HD systems even in developed countries.

So to answer the question: what is the problem in developing countries? There are many answers.

Late ESRD diagnosis or any risk factors can end in ESRD, due to not having a routine checkup in primary health care service.

Incomplete protocols, as already stated, are common in developing countries, making changes to these protocols based on "saving" money only or to provide more medical care to a large number of patients, giving them suboptimal care due to inadequate time for each patient. Because health care providers in developing countries have too many patients, it is not possible to offer optimal service quality.

Unavailability of the adequate equipment.

Not having the right timing between dialysis treatments, and especially between diagnosis and definitive treatment with kidney transplant.

Long waiting lists due to fewer transplant centers for kidney transplantation.

In developing countries, most of the patients are uneducated, or they do not have accurate information about their diseases or their HD route.

In the recommendations given in this chapter, after analyzing the literature and the guidelines for preventing IE in ESRD patients, we summarized the prevention strategies and sought to apply them in any developing country for having less incidence of IE in ESRD patients.

http://dx.doi.org/10.5772/64929

Being part of a health care institution in a developing country, you have to learn how to manage this and other related difficulties. The only method to give a solution to this problem is by analyzing the procedure of other hospitals, either from your region or from other countries, which will give you good arguments for requesting anything missing in your program to provide quality care to their patients. In other words, you have to demonstrate that is cost-effective and it will benefit the patient and the hospital.

Author details

Díaz-García Héctor Rafael[1*], Contreras-de la Torre Nancy Anabel[1], Alemán-Villalobos Alfonso[1], Carrillo-Galindo María de Jesús[1], Gómez-Jiménez Olivia Berenice[1], Esparza-Beléndez Edgar[1], Ramírez-Rosales Gladys Eloísa[2], Portilla-d Buen Eliseo[3] and Arreola-Torres Ramón[1,2,3]

*Address all correspondence to: heradiga@hotmail.com

1 Cardiac Surgery Service, Centro Médico Nacional de Occidente Institutc Mexicano del Seguro Social, Mexico

2 Immunology Laboratory, University Center of Health Sciences, Universidad de Guadalajara, Mexico

3 Surgical Research Division, Biomedical Research Center, Centro Médico Nacional de Occidente Instituto Mexicano del Seguro Social, Mexico

References

[1] Slipczuk L, Codolosa JN, Davila CD, Romero-Corral A, Yun J, Pressman GS, et al. Infective endocarditis epidemiology over five decades: a systematic review. PLoS One. 2013;8(12):e82665.

[2] Bin Abdulhak AA, Baddour LM, Erwin PJ, Hoen B, Chu VH, Mensah GA, et al. Global and regional burden of infective endocarditis, 1990–2010. Global Heart. 2014;9(1):131–143.

[3] Doulton T, Sabharwal N, Cairns HS, Schelenz S, Eykyn S, O'Donnell P, et al. Infective endocarditis in dialysis patients: new challenges and old. Kidney International. 2003;64(2):720–727.

[4] Chang C-F, Kuo BI-T, Chen T-L, Yang W-C, Lee S-D, Lin C-C. Infective endocarditis in maintenance hemodialysis patients: fifteen years' experience in one medical center. Journal of Nephrology. 2004;17(2):228–235.

[5] Nucifora G, Badano LP, Viale P, Gianfagna P, Allocca G, Montanaro D, et al. Infective endocarditis in chronic haemodialysis patients: an increasing clinical challenge. European Heart Journal. 2007;28(19):23072312.

[6] Tleyjeh IM, Abdel-Latif A, Rahbi H, Scott CG, Bailey KR, Steckelberg JM, et al. A systematic review of population-based studies of infective endocarditis. CHEST Journal. 2007;132(3):1025–1035.

[7] Watt G, Lacroix A, Pachirat O, Baggett HC, Raoult D, Fournier P-E, et al. Prospective comparison of infective endocarditis in Khon Kaen, Thailand and Rennes, France. The American Journal of Tropical Medicine and Hygiene. 2015;92(4):871–874.

[8] Kamalakannan D, Pai RM, Johnson LB, Gardin JM, Saravolatz LD. Epidemiology and clinical outcomes of infective endocarditis in hemodialysis patients. The Annals of Thoracic Surgery. 2007;83(6):2081–2086.

[9] Saxena AK, Panhotra BR. Haemodialysis catheter-related bloodstream infections: current treatment options and strategies for prevention. Swiss Medical Weekly. 2005;135(9-10):127–138.

[10] Omoto T, Aoki A, Maruta K, Masuda T. Surgical outcome in hemodialysis patients with active-phase infective endocarditis. Annals of Thoracic and Cardiovascular Surgery. 2016; 22(3):181–185.

[11] Gilmore J. KDOQI clinical practice guidelines and clinical practice recommendations-2006 updates. Nephrology Nursing Journal. 2006;33(5):487.

[12] Hoen B, Paul-Dauphin A, Hestin D, Kessler M. EPIBACDIAL: a multicenter prospective study of risk factors for bacteremia in chronic hemodialysis patients. Journal of the American Society of Nephrology. 1998;9(5):869–876.

[13] Durante-Mangoni E, Bradley S, Selton-Suty C, Tripodi M-F, Barsic B, Bouza E, et al. Current features of infective endocarditis in elderly patients: results of the international collaboration on endocarditis prospective cohort study. Archives of Internal Medicine. 2008;168(19):2095–2103.

[14] Pisoni RL, Young EW, Dykstra DM, Greenwood RN, Hecking E, Gillespie B, et al. Vascular access use in Europe and the United States: results from the DOPPS. Kidney International. 2002;61(1):305–316.

[15] Jones DA, McGill L-A, Rathod KS, Matthews K, Gallagher S, Uppal R, et al. Characteristics and outcomes of dialysis patients with infective endocarditis. Nephron Clinical Practice. 2013;123(3-4):151–156.

[16] Chou M-T, Wang J-J, Wu W-S, Weng S-F, Ho C-H, Lin Z-Z, et al. Epidemiologic features and long-term outcome of dialysis patients with infective endocarditis in Taiwan. International Journal of Cardiology. 2015;179:465–469.

[17] Mylonakis E, Calderwood SB. Infective endocarditis in adults. New England Journal of Medicine. 2001;345(18):1318–1330.

[18] Hoen B. Infective endocarditis: a frequent disease in dialysis patients. Nephrology Dialysis Transplantation. 2004;19(6):1360–1362.

[19] Ferrer C, Almirante B. Venous catheter-related infections. Enferm Infecc Microbiol Clin. 2014;32(2):115–124.

[20] Şimşek-Yavuz S, Şensoy A, Kaşıkçıoğlu H, Çeken S, Deniz D, Yavuz A, et al. Infective endocarditis in Turkey: aetiology, clinical features, and analysis of risk factors for mortality in 325 cases. International Journal of Infectious Diseases. 2015;30:106–114.

[21] Athan E, Chu VH, Tattevin P, Selton-Suty C, Jones P, Naber C, et al. Clinical characteristics and outcome of infective endocarditis involving implantable cardiac devices. JAMA. 2012;307(16):1727–1735.

[22] Heiro M, Helenius H, Mäkilä S, Hohenthal U, Savunen T, Engblom E, et al. Infective endocarditis in a Finnish teaching hospital: a study on 326 episodes treated during 1980–2004. Heart. 2006;92(10):1457–1462.

[23] Nori US, Manoharan A, Thornby JI, Yee J, Parasuraman R, Ramanathan V. Mortality risk factors in chronic haemodialysis patients with infective endocarditis. Nephrology Dialysis Transplantation. 2006;21(8):2184–2190.

[24] Kuo C, Lin J-C, Peng M-Y, Wang N-C, Chang F-Y. Endocarditis: impact of methicillin-resistant *Staphylococcus aureus* in hemodialysis patients and community-acquired infection. Journal of Microbiology, Immunology, and Infection. 2007;40(4):317–324.

[25] Leither MD, Shroff GR, Ding S, Gilbertson DT, Herzog CA. Long-term survival of dialysis patients with bacterial endocarditis undergoing valvular replacement surgery in the United States. Circulation. 2013;128(4):344–351.

[26] Rankin JS, Milford-Beland S, O'Brien SM, Edwards FH, Peterson ED, Glower DD, et al. The risk of valve surgery for endocarditis in patients with dialysis-dependent renal failure. The Journal of Heart Valve Disease. 2007;16(6):617–122; discussion 22.

[27] Spies C, Madison JR, Schatz IJ. Infective endocarditis in patients with end-stage renal disease: clinical presentation and outcome. Archives of Internal Medicine. 2004;164(1): 71–75.

[28] Thourani VH, Sarin EL, Keeling WB, Kilgo PD, Guyton RA, Dara AB, et al. Long-term survival for patients with preoperative renal failure undergoing bioprosthetic or mechanical valve replacement. The Annals of Thoracic Surgery. 2011;91(4):1127–1134.

[29] Pronovost P, Needham D, Berenholtz S, Sinopoli D, Chu H, Cosgrove S, et al. An intervention to decrease catheter-related bloodstream infections in the ICU. New England Journal of Medicine. 2006;355(26):2725–2732.

[30] Chaiyakunapruk N, Veenstra DL, Lipsky BA, Saint S. Chlorhexidine compared with povidone-iodine solution for vascular catheter–site care: a meta-analysis. Annals of Internal Medicine. 2002;136(11):792–801.

[31] Chaiyakunapruk N, Veenstra DL, Lipsky BA, Sullivan SD, Saint S. Vascular catheter site care: the clinical and economic benefits of chlorhexidine gluconate compared with povidone iodine. Clinical Infectious Diseases. 2003;37(6):764–771.

[32] Martínez MP, Lerma FÁ, Badía MR, Gil CL, Pueyo ML, Tobajas CD, et al. Prevention of bacteremia related with ICU catheters by multifactorial intervention: A report of the pilot study. Med Intensiva. 2010;34(9):581–589.

Chapter 8

Septic Embolism: A Potentially Devastating Complication of Infective Endocarditis

Thomas R. Wojda, Kristine Cornejo, Andrew Lin,
Anthony Cipriano, Sudip Nanda, Jose D. Amortegui,
Barbara T. Wojda and Stanislaw P. Stawicki

Additional information is available at the end of the chapter

http://dx.doi.org/10.5772/64931

Abstract

Infective endocarditis is associated with significant cardiac and noncardiac morbidity. Among many complications, septic embolism has the potential of causing devastating sequelae and even life-threatening clinical situations. This dreaded clinico-pathologic entity is characterized by its heterogeneous presentation and the ability to affect various body systems and organs. Septic emboli to the brain, kidneys, spleen, and the pulmonary system constitute the vast majority of metastatic infections. However, other organ systems can also be affected. This chapter provides an overview of septic embolism associated with infective endocarditis, focusing on key diagnostic and therapeutic considerations in the most commonly seen and clinically relevant scenarios.

Keywords: endocarditis, infective endocarditis, septic embolism, diagnosis, treatment

1. Introduction

The importance of septic embolism (SE) associated with infective endocarditis (IE) is both under-appreciated and under-stated [1, 2]. In one large series, systemic arterial embolization or septic pulmonary infarction occurred in approximately 33% and 11% of cases, respectively [1]. Although mortality attributable to IE can exceed 30% [1, 3], it is even higher among patients who experienced SE events [4]. Accurate and timely identification of IE and SE is of critical importance because the presence and type of SE is one of the most important factors taken into consideration when formulating a treatment strategy. Sound clinical judgment and a high index of suspicion are required as the diagnosis of IE and SE is not based on a single test but rather on the combination of clinical findings and diagnostic studies. Microbiologic studies guide antimicrobial therapy. Advanced imaging, including computed tomography (CT) and magnetic resonance imaging (MRI), is used to identify both the extent and location(s) of postembolic infarcts or abscesses. Surgical management, both cardiac and noncardiac, is beyond the scope of the current chapter and is discussed elsewhere in this comprehensive textbook.

2. Infective endocarditis and septic embolism: general clinical, diagnostic and treatment considerations

2.1. General clinical and microbiological considerations

The estimated crude annual incidence of IE is approximately 1 case per 33,000 population, with peak incidence among men between the ages of 70 and 80 years (approximately 1 in 6,900) [1]. Infective endocarditis is a predominantly male disease (50–65% patients) with mean age at the time of presentation between 52 and 63 years, depending on the causative microorganism [1, 3]. Major risk factors for IE include underlying heart disease, cardiac surgery and interventional procedures, prosthetic valve, intravenous drug use, immunosuppression, dental infections, and previous infective endocarditis [1, 3, 5]. Alimentary, genitourinary, respiratory tract, orthopedic, and skin infections, as well as pregnancy-related infection events have also been associated with IE, although far less commonly [3, 6]. Mortality ranges between 6% and 30%, again depending on patient factors and the microorganism(s) involved [1, 3]. Of note, mortality rate was noted to be higher (20%) among patients with IE who experienced embolic or "metastatic" events when compared to individuals without such occurrences (12%) [4].

Clinical presentation of IE involves the development of fever in >90% of cases, with approximately one out of three affected patients experiencing congestive heart failure [1]. Heart murmurs can be present, but may be more reflective of primary valvular disease rather than IE itself [7]. Elevated serum creatinine suggesting renal failure may be present in >25% of cases, and approximately 10% of patients develop septic shock [1]. Rarely, associated life-threatening events such as cardiac tamponade have been reported [8]. According to large clinical series on IE, the most commonly encountered bacteria include *Staphylococci* (19–29% cases), *Streptococci* (44–48%), *Enterococci* (8–19%), Gram-negative organisms, (5–7%), polymicrobial occurrences (0.7–3%), with 5–10% of cases having no microorganisms identified (also known as "culture negative" endocarditis) [1, 3]. Of importance, nosocomial/iatrogenic cases of IE are more likely to be associated with staphylococcal infection when compared to community-acquired IE (35% versus 21%, respectively) [1].

2.2. Pathophysiologic considerations

Septic embolism is most commonly associated with IE, septic thrombophlebitis, periodontal and various systemic infections, as well as central venous catheter and implanted device infections [2]. The combination of aging population, implantable device miniaturization, and the emergence of multi-morbidity have all synergistically contributed to the increased risk of both IE and SE [2, 9]. Thrombogenic characteristics associated with intravascular infections, combined with the relative lack of antibiotic efficacy to clear bloodstream infections, result in elevated risk of SE [10]. According to Millaire et al. [4], embolic events may occur in >50% of IE cases. Fortunately, such events are not associated with significant attributable mortality when properly managed [4]. Further focusing on the cardiac etiology of SE, one of the largest series reported that embolization to the central nervous system was seen in approximately 20% cases of mitral valve IE, 15% cases of aortic valve IE, and 18% combined cases of aortic and mitral IE [1]. When examining right-sided endocarditis, 68% of cases were associated with pulmonary embolization [1]. Finally, it is important to recognize that IE is distinct from nonbacterial thrombotic endocarditis—a pathologic entity that can also result in distal embolization and is beyond the scope of the current chapter [11].

2.3. Septic embolization by anatomic location

When examining the anatomic distribution of nonpulmonary SE in the setting of IE, the most commonly affected organs and organ systems included the central nervous system (48–65%), extremities (30%), spleen (19–32%), and kidney (6–14%) [1, 4, 12]. Less commonly affected structures/organs included the lung (14%), coronary vessels (6%), the liver (3–11%), bone and joint structures (11%), iliac arterial system (6%), and mesenteric arteries (3%) [1, 2, 4]. From anatomic standpoint, a special and more "diffuse" category of embolic events includes musculoskeletal manifestations, which are thought to occur in as many as 44% of cases of SE [13]. Due to their self-limiting nature and nonspecific manifestations (e.g., arthralgias, myalgias, back pain, arthritis), this category of events is often under-reported and tends to be

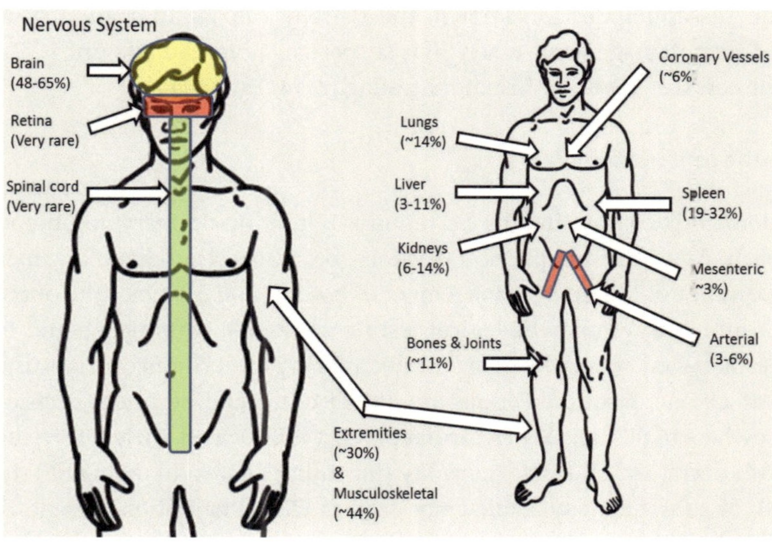

Figure 1. Diagram showing the anatomic distribution of septic emboli in the setting of infectious endocarditis. Compiled from multiple literature sources [1, 2, 4, 12–14].

neglected [14]. **Figure 1** summarizes the anatomic distribution of septic emboli in the setting of IE [1, 2, 4, 12–14]. Of note, anatomic distribution of septic emboli associated with infective endocarditis (48–65% cerebral, 35–52% noncerebral [1, 2, 4]) approximates that of valvular atrial fibrillation (56–63% cerebral, 38–44% noncerebral [15, 16]) suggesting that structural anatomic factors play a role in the pathophysiology of emboli originating from cardiac valves [16–18].

2.4. Diagnostic considerations

Diagnosis of SE requires high index of clinical suspicion, combined with accurate identification and recognition of IE as a source. In the setting of native heart valves, trans-thoracic echocardiography (TTE) should be performed as an initial screening test [19]. If results of the TTE are negative, IE can usually be ruled out if Duke criteria suggest low probability [20, 21]. However, if Duke criteria suggest high suspicion of IE, or if TTE is positive or suspicious for IE, or the patient has a prosthetic valve, the next diagnostic step should be the performance of trans-esophageal echocardiography (TEE) [7, 19–21]. If the TEE is positive, the diagnosis is confirmed. However, if negative, the test can be repeated in 1–2 weeks if clinical suspicion continues to be high [19]. If the above diagnostic steps continue to produce negative results, alternative diagnosis should be entertained.

Multiple, repeated blood culture determinations are often required to identify the causative organism. Although microbiological studies provide critical information regarding targeted antibiotic therapy in IE, results are not always immediately available or universally accurate [22, 23]. Among more recent developments, real-time polymerase chain reaction (PCR) is more sensitive and specific in addition to providing clinically relevant results quickly [24]. Initial antimicrobial coverage should be broad, and once the involved microorganism is identified and antibiotic susceptibilities are known, the therapy can be appropriately narrowed to optimize long-term management. When SE is suspected, advanced imaging (CT and/or MRI) constitutes the cornerstone of confirmatory testing [2, 14, 25, 26].

2.5. Therapeutic considerations

Infective endocarditis complicated by SE requires a multidisciplinary, multimodality therapeutic approach. As outlined in previous sections, broad-spectrum antibiotic management is the most important initial step in management of both IE and SE. Once the offending microorganism is confirmed by microbiological testing, antibiotic coverage should be narrowed according to established sensitivity data. The decision to proceed with cardiac surgical therapy of IE is a complex one, most indications are not absolute, and pertinent decision-making is discussed elsewhere in this text. When cardiac surgery is indicated, early intervention has been associated with decreased all-cause mortality (including deaths following SE) due largely to the lower risk of subsequent systemic embolization [27]. When SE is present, the type and location of emboli guides the treatment strategy. Other surgical and interventional procedures may be utilized to treat complications resulting from SE, including vascular or endovascular interventions for arterial aneurysms [2, 28, 29], percutaneous drainage of abscesses [2], or organ resections (i.e., splenectomy or bowel resection) for infarctions and/or refractory infections [30, 31].

3. Septic emboli to central nervous system

Neurologic complications are a hallmark of left-sided IE and contribute to its unfavorable prognosis [32, 33]. The reported incidence of SE is likely underestimated [4, 34]. In the absence of abnormal intracardiac communication, neurological symptoms develop secondary to emboli originating from left-sided valvular vegetations (**Figure 2**) [1]. Less commonly, neurologic complications can also occur in cases of right-sided endocarditis with patent foramen ovale or other atrial septal defects [35]. A major risk factor for SE to the central nervous system is the delay or lack of appropriate antibiotic therapy [36]. In one study, the incidence of stroke decreased from 4.82 per 1000 patient-days to 1.71 per 1000 patient-days between the first and second weeks of appropriate antimicrobial therapy, respectively [37]. Other risk factors for septic cerebral embolism include vegetation size >10 mm, mobile and multiple vegetations, mitral and/or aortic valve endocarditis, preoperative empiric antibiotic therapy, annular abscess, anticoagulant therapy at the time of IE diagnosis, and the causative organism being *Staphylococcus aureus* [37–43]. Of note, SE to the spleen and kidneys commonly co-occur in patients with cerebral emboli [39].

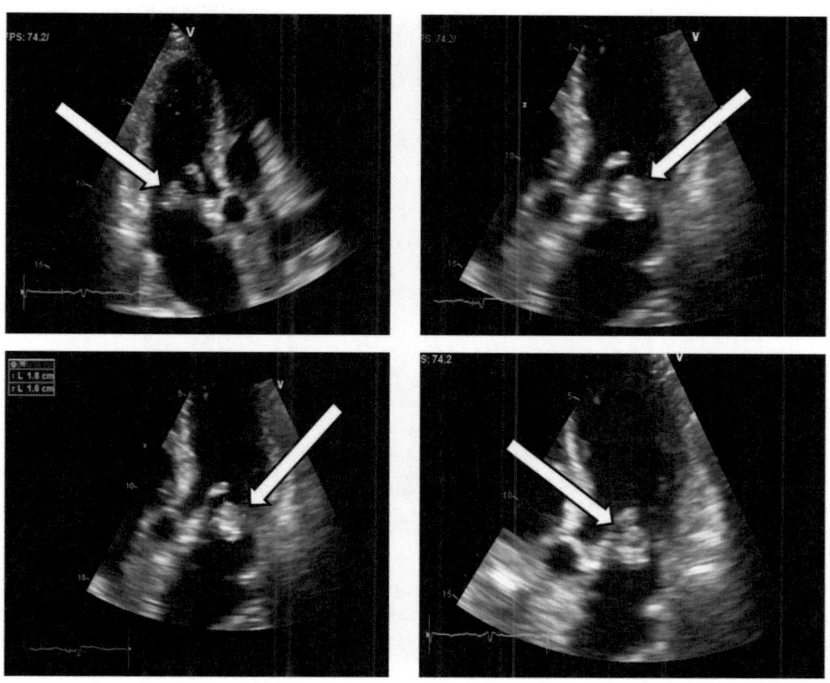

Figure 2. Echocardiography showing large (1.8 × 1.6 cm) mitral valve vegetation (arrows).

Clinical manifestations may include ischemic stroke (**Figure 3**), transient ischemic attack (TIA), cerebral hemorrhage, meningitis, brain abscess, encephalopathy, and mycotic aneurysms [38, 39, 42, 44, 45]. Taken together, these complications often occur early (within the first 7 days of IE) and negatively impact patient outcomes [46]. Among all neurologic manifestations of IE, ischemic stroke and TIA are the most common (16–50% of all occurrences) [38, 39, 44, 45, 47–49]. In approximately 70% of patients with SE of the central nervous system, the middle cerebral artery distribution is involved [38, 44]. Focal neurological symptoms (hemiparesis, facial droop, diplopia, aphasia, vertigo) are present in approximately 40% of affected patients, and nonfocal presentations (headaches, seizures, altered mental status) occur in approximately one-third of cases, with roughly one in five patients remaining asymptomatic [40]. Evaluation should include MRI with and without gadolinium, or CT with and without contrast if MRI is not possible. Vascular imaging should be performed routinely, and CTA or MRA is probably sufficient for screening, with catheter angiography reserved for cases where a mycotic aneurysm was noted and in those patients with an acute brain hemorrhage [50].

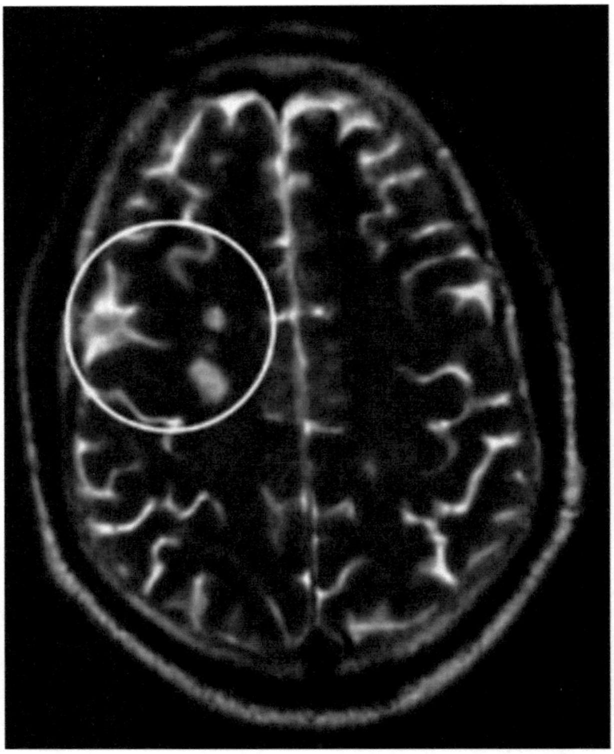

Figure 3. Magnetic resonance imaging (MRI) showing septic embolus to the brain. Source: Stawicki et al. [2]. Used under the terms of the Creative Commons Attribution-Noncommercial-Share Alike 3.0 Unported, which permits unrestricted use, distribution, and reproduction in any medium, provided the original work is properly cited.

A relatively less common manifestation of SE associated with IE is bacterial meningitis, usually presenting with fever, neck stiffness, and altered mental status [51]. The most common causative bacterial species are *Streptococcus pneumoniae* (54%) and *Staphylococcus aureus* (33%) [51]. The diagnosis is confirmed via cerebrospinal fluid analysis, and management requires long-term antibiotic administration and control of the septic source [44, 51].

In addition to being associated with worse clinical outcomes, neurologic complications of SE often force the alteration in therapeutic plans for IE, including the timing/type of operative intervention and the duration of antibiotic treatment [42, 46–49]. Neurological complications negatively impact clinical outcomes, with mortality as high as 45% (compared to 24% in patients who did not experience neurologic sequelae) [43]. Cerebral hemorrhage and moderate-to-severe ischemic events are the main determinants of mortality [43]. Early and appropriate antibiotic therapy remains the cornerstone of IE management and a major preventive strategy to reduce SE to the brain [52]. Although thrombolysis has been traditionally contraindicated for ischemic stroke in the setting of IE due to the risk of massive cerebral hemorrhage [53], some authors have reported good outcomes with thrombolytic therapy in selected cases [44, 54]. Having said that, rates of intracerebral hemorrhage following thrombolysis in such circumstances may be as high as 20% [55].

The use anticoagulation may increase the risk of cerebral hemorrhage without appreciable reduction in the incidence of embolic events, and, as of now, there is no evidence to support this practice [43]. Likewise, antiplatelet agents (including aspirin) were not found to be beneficial in preventing the occurrence of embolic events in a double-blinded, placebo controlled trial [56]. It is recommended to discontinue anticoagulation for at least 2 weeks in patients with IE who develop central nervous system embolic complications regardless of the other indications for anticoagulation, including the presence of mechanical heart valves. The final decision regarding anticoagulation and antiplatelet therapy should be made by a multidisciplinary team including cardiologist, cardiac surgeon, and neurologist [57, 58].

Although uncommon, intracranial mycotic aneurysms are among the most dreaded complications of IE with mortality as high of 16–30% in unruptured cases and 49–80% in ruptured ones [58, 59]. The presentation is variable, with some patients remaining asymptomatic while others developing focal neurologic signs, meningitis, subarachnoid, or intraventricular hemorrhage [58]. Approximately one in five patients may have multiple aneurysmal lesions [60]. Unruptured mycotic aneurysms should be serially monitored and treated conservatively with antibiotic therapy [61]. The treatment of a ruptured cerebral mycotic aneurysm depends on its location, as well as the presence or absence of any associated mass effect [61, 62].

Indications for valvular surgical intervention include, but are not limited to: new severe valvular regurgitation, congestive heart failure, large vegetation (>10 mm), abscess formation, persistently positive blood cultures or emboli despite appropriate antibiotic therapy, prosthetic valve dehiscence, or the presence of highly resistant organisms [63, 64]. Although most patients continue to have an indication for valve surgery after a cerebral SE [47], the timing of cardiac surgery is controversial because the hemorrhagic conversion of an ischemic brain lesion in the setting of intraoperative anticoagulation can be devastating [65–67]. The traditional recommendation is to postpone cardiac surgery for at least 4 weeks [65–67]. The relatively uncommon nature of hemorrhagic conversion of preoperative brain lesions has led some to consider earlier operative therapy in acute IE, hoping to prevent deaths that otherwise would have occurred during the 1 month delay, as well as reducing further embolic events that can cause permanent disability [39]. As a result, evidence is emerging that early operative treatment for patients with nonhemorrhagic cerebral embolic events does not lead to worse outcomes. In a recent report, 198 patients undergoing valve replacement following cerebral infarction were analyzed with 58 undergoing early surgery (1–7 days) and 140 undergoing late surgery (>7 days). There was no survival benefit in delaying otherwise indicated surgery for IE among patients with cerebral SE [68]. Another retrospective study reviewed operative results of 308 patients with IE, finding no difference in key outcomes (postoperative stroke, 30-day mortality, long-term survival) when comparing patients with cerebral SE undergoing early surgery (<14 days) to patients undergoing surgery for IE without cerebral complications [40]. However, some authors report that early cardiac surgery is associated with neurological complications [43]. Both the American Heart Association and The Society of Thoracic Surgeons workforce on evidence-based surgery report that it is probably safe to proceed with an early operation in patients with small ischemic infarction, while delaying a surgery for 2–4 weeks might be preferred for those with a large ischemic infarction or a hemorrhagic event, respectively. In those with worsening cardiac function, recurrent stroke, uncontrolled infection or recurrent emboli, a delay of less than 4 weeks may be reasonable [50, 58].

4. Septic embolism to the kidneys

Despite numerous case reports, available clinical data on SE to the kidneys continue to be limited [2, 69–71]. Embolic events associated with IE involve kidneys in 6–14% cases (**Figure 1**) and exhibit highly variable pattern of presentation [2, 69]. Most patients complain of an acute onset of abdominal, flank, or back pain. The pain is typically constant. Approximately half of reported cases present with fever and vomiting. Acute secondary hypertension from renin release due to decreased arterial perfusion may be seen. Laboratory findings may include leukocytosis, proteinuria, hematuria, elevated levels of lactate dehydrogenase, serum glutamic-oxaloacetic transaminase, serum glutamic-pyruvic transaminase, and alkaline phosphatase [70]. Potential complications of septic emboli include hematuria, glomerulonephritis, or infarction leading to loss of renal function. Three types of severe renal manifestations may be seen: renal infarcts, focal "embolic" glomerulonephritis, and acute diffuse glomerulonephritis [72]. Renal loss due to embolic occlusion of the renal artery has been reported [71]. Of interest, localized renal infarcts were found in over 30% of necropsy samples, with more than half attributable to SE in patients infected with *Staphylococcus aureus* [69]. Renal SE and infarction may be associated with concurrent embolic events to other organs (**Figure 4**) [73]. In one reported case, renal infarction was found in conjunction with SE to the coronary arteries and the spleen [74]. In another case, multiple acute SE infarcts due to Gram-positive aortic valve IE were found in the brain, spleen, kidneys, and the intestine [75]. Treatment is usually supportive, consisting of systemic antibiotics, renal replacement therapy (if indicated) [69], and only rarely involves percutaneous or open procedural interventions [14, 76]. Preservation of renal function is the primary goal.

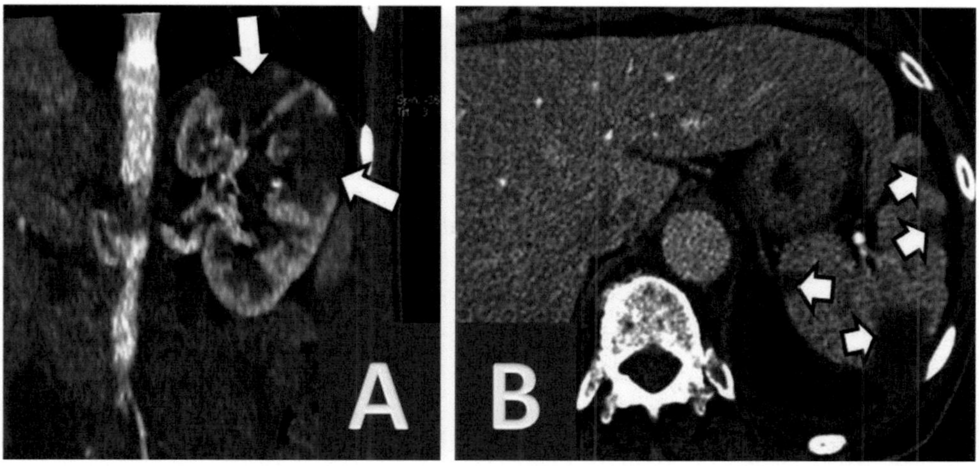

Figure 4. The presence of simultaneous renal (A) and splenic (B) infarctions secondary to septic embolism. Source: Modified from Grob et al. [73]. Used under the terms of the Creative Commons Attribution License (http://creativecommons.org/licenses/by/2.0), which permits unrestricted use, distribution, and reproduction in any medium, provided the original work is properly cited.

5. Septic embolization to spleen

Splenic involvement is often seen in the setting of left-sided valvular vegetations from IE [12]. The two primary manifestations are splenic infarction (most common) and splenic abscess. Although often asymptomatic, splenic infarct may be associated with acute abdominal (usually left upper quadrant) pain and can be complicated by abscess formation (the primary source of subsequent morbidity and mortality) [12, 77]. Splenic abscess formation is due to hematogeneous spread from a distant source of infection, with IE being associated with up to two-thirds of such instances, either via bacteremic seeding or direct embolization of infected valvular debris [78, 79].

In one study, splenic infarcts were found in 19% of cases of IE, including asymptomatic cases identified on CT examination [12]. Streptococci and staphylococci are among the most common offending microorganisms, accounting for >80% of cases [4, 12]. While *Streptococcus viridans* and *Staphylococcus aureus* are frequently encountered, other bacterial species including *K. pneumoniae, S. epidermidis,* and *P. mirabilis* have been described in this setting [79].

Because mortality associated with splenic abscess is high, prompt and appropriate therapy is critical. Management includes antibiotics based on microbial sensitivity, image-guided aspiration or drainage, and surgical intervention by splenectomy (open or laparoscopic) in selected cases [80–83]. Early detection may help reduce the need for surgical intervention. Although the identification of SE to the spleen does not constitute a surgical indication, the presence of an abscess refractory to nonoperative approaches (e.g., antibiotics with or without percutaneous drainage), uncontained abscess rupture, or the presence of vascular complications (e.g., pseudoaneurysm or a large infarction) should prompt the consideration of splenectomy [84–87]. Likewise, refractory pain may also constitute a surgical indication (or be a clinical warning sign of one of the above complications) [80, 87, 88]. The decision to operate in the setting of therapeutic uncertainty should be considered in the context of the simultaneous presence of any other relative indications, risks, and benefits. The diagnosis of splenic infarct is not a contraindication for a cardiac operation when such intervention is indicated. The situation is not as clear in the presence of a splenic abscess. In most cases, it is preferable to perform splenectomy prior to valve surgery in order to prevent re-infection of the valve prosthesis or annuloplasty ring [58, 89]. Combined cardiac procedure and splenectomy has been reported with good outcomes [90].

6. Septic emboli to mesenteric vasculature

Septic embolization to the mesenteric vessels is a serious, potentially life-threatening complication of IE [4]. Small valvular vegetations can break off, enter the circulation, and become lodged in the mesentric arteries, endangering blood supply to the small intestine and colon [91, 92]. Compared to other organ systems affected by metastatic or embolic events of IE, mesenteric embolization is relatively rare, constituting approximately 3% of SE [2]. However, general surgeons must consider this entity on their differential list of causes leading to acute bowel ischemia. In terms of vascular distribution, the inferior mesenteric artery (IMA) involvement is much less common than SE to the superior mesenteric artery (SMA, approximately 3% versus <1%, respectively) [93]. Clinical indications for operative abdominal intervention following mesenteric SE are similar to those for other acute abdominal emergencies and have been discussed elsewhere [94, 95].

Septic embolism involving the mesenteric vessels can also be associated with mycotic aneurysms [96]. Pathophysiology involves embolization of small valvular vegetation fragments to the arterial vasa vasorum or the intraluminal space with subsequent extension of the infection through the intima and outward through the media of the vessel wall [58, 97]. This process gradually weakens the arterial wall, resulting in pathologic dilation and pseudoaneurysm formation [58]. Depending on the anatomic characteristics of the pseudoaneurysm, and the presence versus absence of associated distal embolization/thrombosis, management may include resection or vascular bypass of the lesion [98]. Inherent to the nature of pseudoaneurysms secondary to SE, high complication rate and/or mortality may be encountered [98].

In one unusual case, *Streptococcus bovis* endocarditis was reported to be associated with SE to the superior mesenteric artery (SMA) resulting in a mycotic aneurysm. Computed tomography (CT) imaging demonstrated a saccular aneurysm of the SMA and follow-up angiography showed evidence of SE to the left femoral artery [99]. A duplex ultrasound further characterized the femoral artery lesion as an intravascular mass at the left femoral artery bifurcation. Echocardiography confirmed mitral valvular vegetations. The patient underwent surgical resection of the mesenteric aneurysm, embolectomy of the femoral artery, as well as mitral valve replacement procedure [99].

In another report, *Coxiella burnetii* endocarditis led to concurrent SMA embolism and renal infarction. The patient presented with acute abdominal and flank pain, with subsequent CT of the abdomen demonstrating acute infarct of the right kidney and suspected SMA emboli [100]. The patient underwent laparotomy and successful SMA balloon thromboembolectomy. Subsequent TEE demonstrated a heterogeneous, mobile aortic valve mass. The patient was started on triple antibiotic regimen of vancomycin, gentamicin, and ceftriaxone. Subsequent aortic valve replacement was performed using a pericardial valve, with good long-term clinical outcome [100].

7. Right-sided endocarditis and septic pulmonary embolism

Right-sided IE (**Figure 5**) usually manifests as persistent fevers, bacteremia, and multiple septic pulmonary emboli (SPE, **Figure 6**). Isolated pulmonary valve endocarditis accounts for only about 2% of IE cases [101]. Due to its rarity, SPE is often difficult to diagnose due to its nonspecific presentation. In addition to the signs and symptoms of IE, SPE may cause pleuritic chest pain, cough, and/or hemoptysis [102] and may be complicated by pulmonary infarction, abscess, pneumothorax, pulmonary infiltrates, and purulent pulmonary effusion [103–105]. Although rare, right-sided heart failure due to increased pulmonary arterial pressure or severe right-sided valvular regurgitation/obstruction may occur. Historically, SPE was associated with intravenous drug use [106]. However, today the most common clinical risk factors include indwelling intravascular catheters, intravascular devices, and noncardiac sources of sepsis, especially in hospitalized patients [107–110].

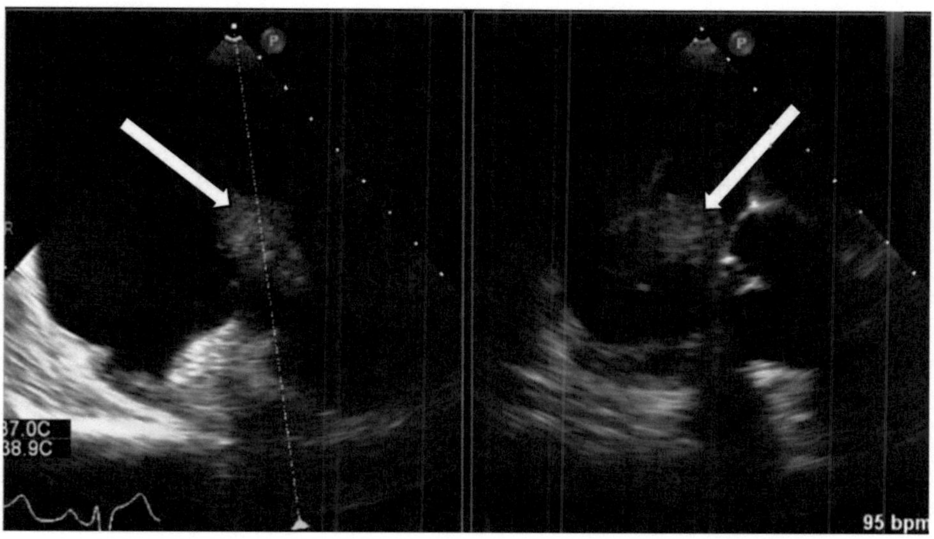

Figure 5. Echocardiographic images of tricuspid valve endocarditis characterized by the presence of a large vegetation (arrows).

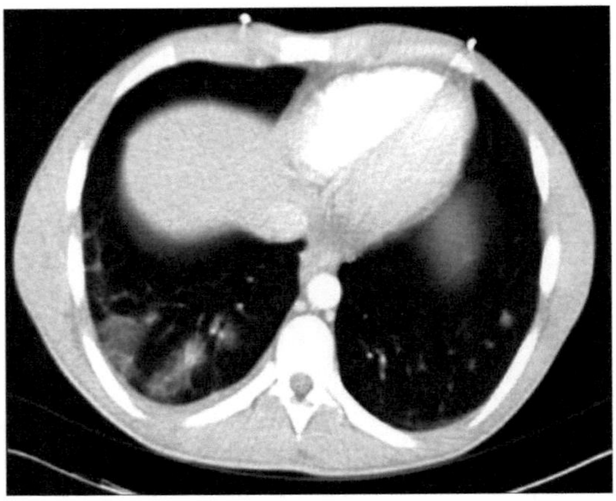

Figure 6. Septic pulmonary emboli associated with tricuspid valve endocarditis due to methicillin-resistant Staphylococcus aureus. Source: Stawicki et al. [2]. Used under the terms of the Creative Commons Attribution-Noncommercial-Share Alike 3.0 Unported, which permits unrestricted use, distribution, and reproduction in any medium, provided the original work is properly cited.

Regarding diagnostic modalities used in the setting of suspected SPE, chest radiography is nonspecific and usually shows poorly marginated peripheral lung nodules, possibly with cavitary features [25]. Computed tomography provides much better image granularity and usually demonstrates bilateral nodules or multifocal infiltrates, often involving peripheral lung zones and associated cavitary lesions [102]. These features, in conjunction with extrapulmonary infection, should raise suspicion of SPE as the underlying cause. The "feeding vessel" sign, or the finding of a vessel which projects into a peripheral lung lesion, is fairly specific for SPE [111, 112]. Patients with SPE and suspected IE should undergo echocardiography to rule out valvular infection and to assess for any associated cardiac complications [113, 114]. TEE is preferred over TTE due to better image resolution and improved diagnostic accuracy for detecting small vegetations, abscesses, and leaflet perforations up to 5 mm in size [113, 114].

A conservative approach is recommended in most patients with right-sided IE because significant majority of the cases will resolve with antimicrobial therapy alone [115, 116]. The role of surgery remains unclear because the presence of SPE and/or recurrent SPE is not an absolute indication for operative intervention. Surgery is usually indicated in cases of persistent sepsis, lack of response to appropriate antimicrobial therapy, right heart failure secondary to severe tricuspid regurgitation, and persistent large vegetation [50, 58, 117, 118]. Thoracoscopy or thoracotomy may be required in complicated cases of SPE (e.g., empyema, pulmonary abscess) [102, 106].

8. Additional considerations and special topics

Majority of the literature on IE and SE is devoted to the most common and clinically relevant presentations, leading to a degree of "neglect" toward the unusual yet still potentially significant complications. In this section, the authors will discuss other, less common manifestations of SE. More specifically, we will focus on septic emboli to various anatomic locations, in decreasing order of incidence.

8.1. Septic emboli to solid abdominal organs

A significant proportion of SE involves abdominal and retroperitoneal solid organs (e.g., liver, spleen, pancreas, kidneys). Emboli to the more commonly affected locations (e.g., spleen and kidney) have been discussed earlier in this manuscript. It is important to remember that septic embolic phenomena tend to simultaneously involve more than one anatomic location, with significant proportion of events being asymptomatic [75, 119]. At times, smaller septic embolic lesions may coalesce to form well-defined abscesses [120]. The next two sections will discuss hepatic and pancreatic SE occurrences.

8.2. Septic embolism to the liver

Liver abscesses due to SE associated with IE are well documented in the medical literature [121]. As outlined above, larger hepatic abscesses may evolve over time from smaller, adjacent microabscesses [120]. Infectious endocarditis should be entertained in the setting of any hepatic abscess of uncertain etiology, with echocardiography undertaken in order to rule out cardiac valvular source [122]. Clinical approach is usually multi-modal, including broad-spectrum antibiotics, endoscopy, percutaneous drainage, and/or surgery [2].

8.3. Septic emboli to the pancreas

Pancreatic septic emboli have been described in the setting of multi-visceral SE [75]. Due to the disproportionate severity of concurrent embolic events, pancreatic SE is likely under-reported and under-appreciated. Clinical presentation of pancreatic SE may resemble that of pancreatitis (e.g., abdominal pain, elevated serum amylase/lipase, leukocytosis, and peri-pancreatic inflammatory changes on advanced imaging) [2]. The range of possible clinical presentations spans from that of self-limited pancreatitis to an overwhelming necrotizing infection. Associated findings may also include vascular abnormalities (e.g., pseudoaneurysms) involving nearby vasculature (i.e., pancreaticoduodenal artery) on advanced imaging [123].

8.4. Coronary septic emboli

Coronary embolization from a septic focus has been relatively well reported in the literature [74, 124] and usually originates from valvular vegetations in the setting of IE [125]. Septic coronary embolism has also been reported to occur intraoperatively during mitral valve surgery performed in the setting of IE [126]. Coronary arterial SE should be entertained in cases of known or suspected left-sided IE and evidence of concurrent acute myocardial ischemia (e.g., abnormal ECG or elevated cardiac enzymes). Echocardiography (preferably TEE) can reliably demonstrate the presence of valvular vegetations, in addition to documenting other changes characteristics of myocardial ischemia [127]. Coronary occlusion secondary to SE can also be confirmed via coronary angiography, with the potential for percutaneous coronary intervention at the same time [128]. Acutely occluded major coronary arteries or branches may require surgical revascularization at the time of valve surgery. Patients with aortic valve endocarditis, in whom preoperative coronary angiography may be contraindicated due to concerns of dislodging debris, may require empiric grafting [2]. An example of a mycotic coronary artery aneurysm associated with IE is shown in **Figure 7**.

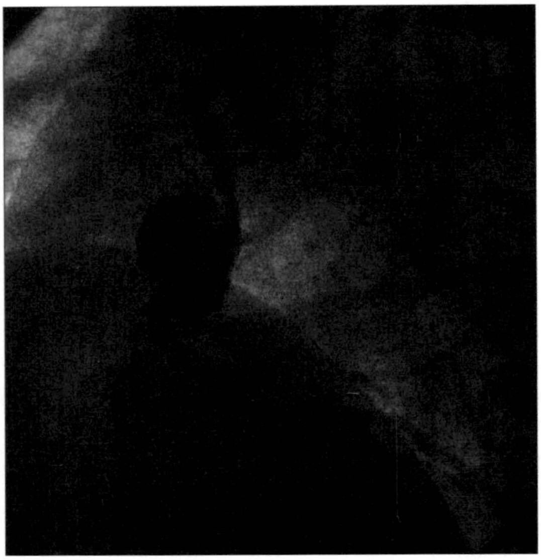

Figure 7. Mycotic aneurysm of the right coronary artery. The patient underwent venous bypass grafting. Source: Stawicki et al. [2]. Used under the terms of the Creative Commons Attribution-Noncommercial-Share Alike 3.0 Unported, which permits unrestricted use, distribution, and reproduction in any medium, provided the original work is properly cited.

8.5. Septic emboli to extremities

Distal septic emboli are well described in the setting of IE [30, 129]. A nontrivial proportion of SE associated with IE requiring valvular replacement affects the extremities, with some patients experiencing multiple embolic events [30, 129]. Clinical manifestations can vary from extremity pain to limb-threatening ischemia [30]. In less severe cases, ischemic symptoms may resolve with anticoagulation and antimicrobial therapy, while in more acute presentations surgical embolectomy or even amputation may be required [30].

8.6. Arterial lesions associated with septic embolism

Secondary arterial changes and associated lesions have been reported in the setting of infectious embolization [75, 130]. Inflammatory changes were noted in the walls of arteries adjacent to an intracranial hematoma following septic embolization [75]. In one instance, brachial artery pseudoaneurysm (**Figure 8**) has been described in the setting of severe prosthetic aortic valve endocarditis [2]. In another case, a ruptured mycotic aortic abdominal aneurysm occurred in a child with SE following the resection of an infected cardiac myxoma [131]. Due to rarity of such arterial lesions and the associated nonspecific clinical presentation(s), it is extremely important to maintain a high index of suspicion when potential infections of arterial structures are identified.

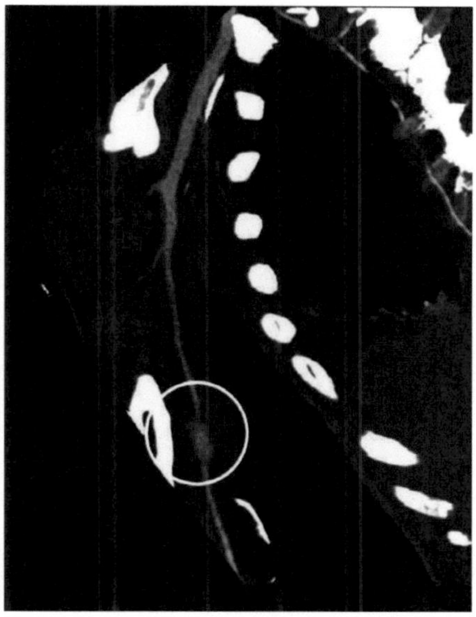

Figure 8. Large (2.5 cm) brachial artery pseudoaneurysm secondary to septic embolization from prosthetic aortic valve endocarditis. Source: Stawicki et al. [2]. Used under the terms of the Creative Commons Attribution-Noncommercial-Share Alike 3.0 Unported, which permits unrestricted use, distribution, and reproduction in any medium, provided the original work is properly cited.

8.7. Uncommon presentations involving the central nervous system

Exceedingly rare, septic embolism may involve the spinal cord and lead to associated spinal cord infarction [132, 133]. In such cases, other organs are likely to become involved as well, including the kidneys and pulmonary circulation [132]. Finally, septic embolism to the retina has been reported in the setting of staphylococcal tricuspid endocarditis in intravenous drug abusers [119].

9. Conclusions

Despite significant evolution of both diagnostic and therapeutic approaches, septic emboli continue to present a formidable challenge to the practicing clinician. In addition to high index of suspicion and early clinical recognition, prompt identification of the offending cardiac source and the institution of immediate goal-directed antibiotic therapy are all critical to successful outcomes. More widespread awareness of risk factors, clinical presentations, and management of SE is needed, with added focus on preventing embolic events and the management of associated complications.

Acknowledgements

The authors like to acknowledge the help of Dr Andrew Halpern and Dr Amitoj Singh for their help with obtaining radiographic and echocardiographic images of infective endocarditis and septic emboli.

Author details

Thomas R. Wojda[1,2], Kristine Cornejo[2,3], Andrew Lin[4], Anthony Cipriano[1], Sudip Nanda[5], Jose D. Amortegui[1,5], Barbara T. Wojda[6] and Stanislaw P. Stawicki[1,2*]

*Address all correspondence to: stanislaw.stawicki@sluhn.org

1 Department of Surgery, St. Luke's University Health Network, Bethlehem, PA, USA

2 Department of Research and Innovation, EW-2 Research Administration, St. Luke's University Health Network, Bethlehem, PA, USA

3 Family Medicine Residency Program, Warren Hospital, St. Luke's University Health Network, Phillipsburg, NJ, USA

4 St. Luke's University Hospital Campus, Temple University School of Medicine, Bethlehem, PA, USA

5 Heart and Vascular Center, St. Luke's University Health Network, Bethlehem, PA, USA

6 Department of Internal Medicine, University of Louisville School of Medicine, Louisville, KY, USA

References

[1] Hoen, B., et al., Changing profile of infective endocarditis: results of a 1-year survey in France. JAMA, 2002. 288(1): p. 75–81.

[2] Stawicki, S.P., et al., Septic embolism in the intensive care unit. Int J Crit Illn Inj Sci, 2013. 3(1): p. 58, doi:10.4103/2229-5151.109423.

[3] Bayliss, R., et al., The microbiology and pathogenesis of infective endocarditis. Br Heart J, 1983. 50(6): p. 513–519.

[4] Millaire, A., et al., Incidence and prognosis of embolic events and metastatic infections in infective endocarditis. Eur Heart J, 1997. 18(4): p. 677–684.

[5] Ward, M. and K.M. Boehm, Pacemaker related infective endocarditis from *Staphylococcus lugdunensis*: A case report. Case Reports in Critical Care, 2013. p. 3, doi: 10.1155/2013/180401

[6] Bayliss, R., et al., The bowel, the genitourinary tract, and infective endocarditis. Br Heart J, 1984. 51(3): p. 339–345.

[7] Erbel, R., et al., Improved diagnostic value of echocardiography in patients with infective endocarditis by transoesophageal approach. A prospective study. Eur Heart J, 1988. 9(1): p. 43–53.

[8] Raizes, E.G., M.B. Livingston, and W.E. Farrar, Fatal cardiac tamponade in a young man with group C streptococcal endocarditis. Am J Med Sci, 1987. 294(5): p. 353–356.

[9] Birriel, T.J., et al., Adverse drug reactions in the era of multi-morbidity and polypharmacy. J Basic Clin Pharm, 2015. 6(4): p. 122–123.

[10] Dickman, F.N. and I.B. Moore, Mycotic aneurysms: a case report of a popliteal mycotic aneurysm. Ann Surg, 1968. 167(4): p. 590–594.

[11] MacDonald, R.A. and S.L. Robbins, The significance of nonbacterial thrombotic endocarditis: an autopsy and clinical study of 78 cases. Ann Intern Med, 1957. 46(2): p. 255–273.

[12] Ting, W., et al., Splenic septic emboli in endocarditis. Circulation, 1990. 82(5 Suppl): p. IV105–IV109.

[13] Churchill, M.A., Jr., J.E. Geraci, and G.G. Hunder, Musculoskeletal manifestations of bacterial endocarditis. Ann Intern Med, 1977. 87(6): p. 754–759.

[14] Colen, T.W., et al., Radiologic manifestations of extra-cardiac complications of infective endocarditis. Eur Radiol, 2008. 18(11): p. 2433–2445.

[15] Szekely, P., Systemic embolism and anticoagulant prophylaxis in rheumatic heart disease. Br Med J, 1964. 1(5392): p. 1209–1212.

[16] Roy, D., et al., Usefulness of anticoagulant therapy in the prevention of embolic complications of atrial fibrillation. Am Heart J, 1986. 112(5): p. 1039–1043.

[17] Hart, R.G., et al., Factors associated with ischemic stroke during aspirin therapy in atrial fibrillation analysis of 2012 participants in the SPAF I–III clinical trials. Stroke, 1999. 30(6): p. 1223–1229.

[18] Fang, M.C., et al., Gender differences in the risk of ischemic stroke and peripheral embolism in atrial fibrillation the anticoagulation and risk factors in atrial fibrillation (ATRIA) study. Circulation, 2005. 112(12): p. 1687–1691.

[19] Motwani, M. Echocardiography in Infective Endocarditis. 2010 [cited 2016 June 18, 2016]; Available from: http://citeseerx.ist.psu.edu/viewdoc/download?doi=10.1.1.662.3802&rep=rep1&type=pdf.

[20] Dodds, G.A., et al., Negative predictive value of the Duke criteria for infective endocarditis. Am J Cardiol, 1996. 77(5): p. 403–407.

[21] Li, J.S., et al., Proposed modifications to the Duke criteria for the diagnosis of infective endocarditis. Clin Infect Dis, 2000. 30(4): p. 633–638.

[22] Durack, D.T., et al., New criteria for diagnosis of infective endocarditis: utilization of specific echocardiographic findings. Am J Med, 1994. 96(3): p. 200–209.

[23] Breitkopf, C., et al., Impact of a molecular approach to improve the microbiological diagnosis of infective heart valve endocarditis. Circulation, 2005. 111(11): p. 1415–1421.

[24] Miller, R.J., et al., Development and evaluation of a novel fast broad-range 16S ribosomal DNA PCR and sequencing assay for diagnosis of bacterial infective endocarditis: multi-year experience in a large Canadian healthcare zone and a literature review. BMC Infect Dis, 2016. 16(1): p. 1.

[25] Huang, R.-M., et al., Septic pulmonary emboli: CT-radiographic correlation. Am J Roentgenol, 1989. 153(1): p. 41–45.

[26] Fatahzadeh, M. and M. Glick, Stroke: epidemiology, classification, risk factors, complications, diagnosis, prevention, and medical and dental management. Oral Surg Oral Med Oral Pathol Oral Radiol Endod, 2006. 102(2): p. 180–191.

[27] Kang, D.-H., Timing of surgery in infective endocarditis. Heart, 2015: http://heart.bmj.com/citmgr?gca=heartjnl%3Bheartjnl-2015-307878v1

[28] McCready, R.A., et al., Infected splenic artery aneurysm with associated splenic abscess formation secondary to bacterial endocarditis: case report and review of the literature. J Vasc Surg, 2007. 45(5): p. 1066–1068.

[29] Hall, C., et al., Life threatening haemorrhage from a mycotic renal pseudoaneurysm treated by segmental renal artery embolisation. Br Med J (Clinical research ed.), 1987. 294(6586): p. 1526.

[30] Kitts, D., F.S. Bongard, and S.R. Klein, Septic embolism complicating infective endocarditis. J Vasc Surg, 1991. 14(4): p. 480–487.

[31] Misawa, S., et al., Septic embolic occlusion of the superior mesenteric artery induced by mitral valve endocarditis. Ann Thorac Cardiovasc Surg, 2011. 17(4): p. 415–417.

[32] Chu, V.H., et al., Early predictors of in-hospital death in infective endocarditis. Circulation, 2004. 109(14): p. 1745–1749.

[33] Heiro, M., et al., Neurologic manifestations of infective endocarditis: a 17-year experience in a teaching hospital in Finland. Arch Intern Med, 2000. 160(18): p. 2781–2787.

[34] Forbes, G.B., Neurologic complications of systemic disease. Postgrad Med, 1954. 15(2): p. 157–162.

[35] Cunha, B.A., M.V. Gill, and J.M. Lazar, Acute infective endocarditis: diagnostic and therapeutic approach. Infect Dis Clin North Am, 1996. 10(4): p. 811–834.

[36] Sonneville, R., et al., Management of neurological complications of infective endocarditis in ICU patients. Ann Intensive Care, 2011. 1(1): p. 10.

[37] Thuny, F., et al., Risk of embolism and death in infective endocarditis: prognostic value of echocardiography: a prospective multicenter study. Circulation, 2005. 112(1): p. 69–75.

[38] Lee, S.J., et al., Clinical significance of cerebrovascular complications in patients with acute infective endocarditis: a retrospective analysis of a 12-year single-center experience. BMC Neurol, 2014. 14: p. 30.

[39] Misfeld, M., et al., Surgery for infective endocarditis complicated by cerebral embolism: a consecutive series of 375 patients. J Thorac Cardiovasc Surg, 2014. 147(6): p. 1837–1844.

[40] Sorabella, R.A., et al., Early operation for endocarditis complicated by preoperative cerebral emboli is not associated with worsened outcomes. Ann Thorac Surg, 2015. 100(2): p. 501–508.

[41] Kim, D.H., et al., Impact of early surgery on embolic events in patients with infective endocarditis. Circulation, 2010. 122(11 Suppl): p. S17–S22.

[42] Sonneville, R., et al., Neurologic complications and outcomes of infective endocarditis in critically ill patients: the ENDOcardite en REAnimation prospective multicenter study. Crit Care Med, 2011. 39(6): p. 1474–1481.

[43] García-Cabrera, E., et al., Neurologic complications of infective endocarditis: risk factors, outcome, and impact of cardiac surgery: a multicenter observational study. Circulation, 2013. 127: p. 2272–2284.doi: 10.1161/CIRCULATIONAHA.112.000813.

[44] Novy, E., et al., Neurological complications of infective endocarditis: new breakthroughs in diagnosis and management. Med Mal Infect, 2013. 43(11–12): p. 443–450.

[45] Duval, X., et al., Effect of early cerebral magnetic resonance imaging on clinical decisions in infective endocarditis: a prospective study. Ann Intern Med, 2010. 152(8): p. 497–504, W175.

[46] Mourvillier, B., et al., Infective endocarditis in the intensive care unit: clinical spectrum and prognostic factors in 228 consecutive patients. Intensive Care Med, 2004. 30(11): p. 2046–2052.

[47] Murdoch, D.R., et al., Clinical presentation, etiology, and outcome of infective endocarditis in the 21st century: the International Collaboration on Endocarditis-Prospective Cohort Study. Arch Intern Med, 2009. 169(5): p. 463–473.

[48] Pruitt, A.A., Neurologic complications of infective endocarditis. Curr Treat Options Neurol, 2013. 15(4): p. 465–476.

[49] Chaudhary, G. and J.D. Lee, Neurologic complications of infective endocarditis. Curr Neurol Neurosci Rep, 2013. 13(10): p. 380.

[50] Byrne, J.G., et al., Surgical management of endocarditis: the society of thoracic surgeons clinical practice guideline. Ann Thorac Surg, 2011. 91(6): p. 2012–2019.

[51] Lucas, M.J., et al., Endocarditis in adults with bacterial meningitis. Circulation, 2013. 127(20): p. 2056–2062.

[52] Habib, G., et al., Guidelines on the prevention, diagnosis, and treatment of infective endocarditis (new version 2009): the Task Force on the Prevention, Diagnosis, and Treatment of Infective Endocarditis of the European Society of Cardiology (ESC). Endorsed by the European Society of Clinical Microbiology and Infectious Diseases (ESCMID) and the International Society of Chemotherapy (ISC) for Infection and Cancer. Eur Heart J, 2009. 30(19): p. 2369–2413.

[53] Derex, L., E. Bonnefoy, and F. Delahaye, Impact of stroke on therapeutic decision making in infective endocarditis. J Neurol, 2010. 257(3): p. 315–321.

[54] Sontineni, S.P., et al., Effectiveness of thrombolytic therapy in acute embolic stroke due to infective endocarditis. Stroke Research and Treatment, 2010. 2010: p. 5, doi: 10.4061/2010/841797

[55] Asaithambi, G., M.M. Adil, and A.I. Qureshi, Thrombolysis for ischemic stroke associated with infective endocarditis: results from the nationwide inpatient sample. Stroke, 2013. 44(10): p. 2917–2919.

[56] Chan, K.-L., et al., A randomized trial of aspirin on the risk of embolic events in patients with infective endocarditis. J Am Coll Cardiol, 2003. 42(5): p. 775–780.

[57] Nishimura, R.A., et al., 2014 AHA/ACC guideline for the management of patients with valvular heart disease: a report of the American College of Cardiology/American Heart Association Task Force on Practice Guidelines. J Am Coll Cardiol, 2014. 63(22): p. e57–e185.

[58] Baddour, L.M., et al., Infective endocarditis in adults: diagnosis, antimicrobial therapy, and management of complications a scientific statement for healthcare professionals from the American Heart Association. Circulation, 2015. 132(15): p. 1435–1486.

[59] Peters, P.J., T. Harrison, and J.L. Lennox, A dangerous dilemma: management of infectious intracranial aneurysms complicating endocarditis. Lancet Infect Dis, 2006. 6(11): p. 742–748.

[60] Clare, C. and D. Barrow, Infectious intracranial aneurysms. Neurosurg Clin N Am, 1992. 3(3): p. 551–566.

[61] Gross, B.A. and A.S. Puri, Endovascular treatment of infectious intracranial aneurysms. Neurosurg Rev, 2013. 36(1): p. 11–19; discussion 19.

[62] Chapot, R., et al., Endovascular treatment of cerebral mycotic aneurysms. Radiology, 2002. 222(2): p. 389–396.

[63] Ramsdale, D.R., T. Elliott, and P. Wright, Guidance on the prophylaxis and treatment of infective endocarditis in adults.

[64] Kang, N. and W. Smith, Surgical management of infective endocarditis. Circulation, 1965. 13: p. 450.

[65] Horstkotte, D., et al., Guidelines on prevention, diagnosis and treatment of infective endocarditis executive summary. Eur Heart J, 2004. 25(3): p. 267–276.

[66] Angstwurm, K., et al., Timing the valve replacement in infective endocarditis involving the brain. J Neurol, 2004. 251(10): p. 1220–1226.

[67] Rossi, M., et al., What is the optimal timing for surgery in infective endocarditis with cerebrovascular complications? Interact Cardiovasc Thorac Surg, 2012. 14(1): p. 72–80.

[68] Barsic, B., et al., Influence of the timing of cardiac surgery on the outcome of patients with infective endocarditis and stroke. Clin Infect Dis, 2013. 56(2): p. 209–217.

[69] Majumdar, A., et al., Renal pathological findings in infective endocarditis. Nephrol Dial Transplant, 2000. 15(11): p. 1782–1787.

[70] Lessman, R.K., et al., Renal artery embolism: clinical features and long-term follow-up of 17 cases. Ann Intern Med, 1978. 89(4): p. 477–482.

[71] Allen, A.W. and M.T. Warren, Bacterial endocarditis presenting with unilateral renal artery occlusion treated with the Rinspirator Thrombus Removal System rinsing and thrombectomy device and suction thrombectomy. J Vasc Surg, 2009. 49(6): p. 1585–1587.

[72] Mittal, B., Renal lesions in infective endocarditis (an autopsy study of 55 cases). J Postgrad Med, 1987. 33(4): p. 193.

[73] Grob, A., et al., Cardiac multidetector computed tomography in infective endocarditis: a pictorial essay. Insights Imaging, 2014. 5(5): p. 559–570, doi:10.1007/s13244-014-0353-1.

[74] Caraballo, V., Fatal myocardial infarction resulting from coronary artery septic embolism after abortion: unusual cause and complication of endocarditis. Ann Emerg Med, 1997. 29(1): p. 175–177.

[75] Hart, R.G., K. Kagan-Hallet, and S.E. Joerns, Mechanisms of intracranial hemorrhage in infective endocarditis. Stroke, 1987. 18(6): p. 1048–1056.

[76] Townell, N.J., et al., Community-associated methicillin-resistant staphylococcus aureus endocarditis 'down under': case series and literature review. Scand J Infect Dis, 2012. 44(7): p. 536–540.

[77] Beeson, M.S., Splenic infarct presenting as acute abdominal pain in an older patient. J Emerg Med, 1996. 14(3): p. 319–322.

[78] Farres, H., et al., Management of splenic abscess in a critically ill patient. Surg Laparosc Endosc Percutan Tech, 2004. 14(2): p. 49–52.

[79] Elasfar, A., et al., Splenic abscess associated with infective endocarditis; Case series. J Saudi Heart Assoc, 2015. 27(3): p. 210–215.

[80] Millaire, A., et al., Incidence and prognosis of embolic events and metastatic infections in infective endocarditis. Eur Heart J, 1997. 18(4): p. 677–684.

[81] Simsir, S.A., et al., Staged laparoscopic splenectomy and valve replacement in splenic abscess and infective endocarditis. Ann Thorac Surg, 2003. 75(5): p. 1635–1637.

[82] Green, B.T., Splenic abscess: report of six cases and review of the literature. Am Surg, 2001. 67(1): p. 80–85.

[83] Carbonell, A.M., et al., Laparoscopic splenectomy for splenic abscess. Surg Laparosc Endosc Percutan Tech, 2004. 14(5): p. 289–291.

[84] Nores, M., et al., The clinical spectrum of splenic infarction. Am Surg, 1998. 64(2): p. 182.

[85] Ooi, L.L.P. and S.S. Leong, Splenic abscesses from 1987 to 1995. Am J Surg, 1997. 174(1): p. 87–93.

[86] Narra, R.K. and M.V. Jehendran, Ruptured splenic abscess causing pneumoperitoneum: a rare cause revisited. BMJ Case Rep, 2015. 2015: p. bcr2014209055.

[87] Uranüs, S. and O. Alimoglu, Splenic abscess and infarction–rare events for which surgery is mandatory. Eur Surg, 2003. 35(6): p. 326–326. http://link.springer.com/article/10.1007%2Fs10353-003-0039-2?LI=true

[88] Pothula, V., et al., Splenic syndrome: a rare indication for splenectomy. Mil Med, 2008. 173(12): p. 1233–1237.

[89] Ebels, J., et al., Splenic abscess complicating infective endocarditis: three case reports. Acta Chir Belg, 2007. 107(6): p. 720–723.

[90] Akhyari, P., et al., Is simultaneous splenectomy an additive risk factor in surgical treatment for active endocarditis? Langenbeck's Arch Surg, 2012. 397(8): p. 1261–1266.

[91] Murray, D.G., Embolism in peripheral arteries. Can Med Assoc J, 1936. 35(1): p. 61.

[92] Byard, R.W., Acute mesenteric ischaemia and unexpected death. J Forensic Leg Med, 2012. 19(4): p. 185–190.

[93] Kirkwood, M.L., et al., Mycotic inferior mesenteric artery aneurysm secondary to native valve endocarditis caused by coagulase-negative Staphylococcus. Ann Vasc Surg, 2014. 28(5): p. 1312. e13–e15.

[94] Schwartz, J., et al., Gastrointestinal complications in cardiothoracic surgery: a synopsis. Principles and Practice of Cardiothoracic Surgery, InTech, Rijeka, Croatia, 2013.

[95] Endean, E.D., et al., Surgical management of thrombotic acute intestinal ischemia. Ann Surg, 2001. 233(6): p. 801–808.

[96] Pasha SF, Gloviczki P, Stanson AW, Kamath PS. Splanchnic artery aneurysms. In Mayo Clinic Proceedings 2007 Apr 30. 82(4): p. 472–479). Elsevier: Rochester.

[97] Suliman, F.A., Infective endocarditis clinical presentation and outcome in Sudanese patients. 2015, UOFK.

[98] Teixeira, P.G., et al., Infective endocarditis associated superior mesenteric artery pseudoaneurysm. Ann Vasc Surg, 2014. 28(6): p. 1563. e1–e5.

[99] Chai, H.-T., et al., Infective endocarditis caused by *Streptococcus bovis* complicated by a superior mesenteric artery mycotic aneurysm and systemic septic emboli in a patient with colon diverticulitis. Int J Infec Dis, 2010. 14: p. e317–e318.

[100] Raizada, A., N. Apte, and S. Pham, Q fever endocarditis presenting with superior mesenteric artery embolism and renal infarction. Tex Heart Inst J, 2016. 43(1): p. 91–93.

[101] Cassling, R.S., W.C. Rogler, and B.M. McManus, Isolated pulmonic valve infective endocarditis: a diagnostically elusive entity. Am Heart J, 1985. 109(3): p. 558–567.

[102] Cook, R.J., et al., Septic pulmonary embolism: presenting features and clinical course of 14 patients. CHEST J, 2005. 128(1): p. 162–166.

[103] Miró, J.M., A. del Río, and C.A. Mestres, Infective endocarditis and cardiac surgery in intravenous drug abusers and HIV-1 infected patients. Cardiol Clin, 2003. 21(2): p. 167–184.

[104] Chambers, H.F., O.M. Korzeniowski, and M.A. Sande, *Staphylococcus aureus* endocarditis: clinical manifestations in addicts and nonaddicts. Medicine, 1983. 62(3): p. 170–177.

[105] Rossi, S.E., P.C. Goodman, and T. Franquet, Nonthrombotic pulmonary emboli. Am J Roentgenol, 2000. 174(6): p. 1499–1508.

[106] MacMillan, J., S. Milstein, and P. Samson, Clinical spectrum of septic pulmonary embolism and infarction. J Thorac Cardiovasc Surg, 1978. 75(5): p. 670–679.

[107] Karchmer, A.W. and D.L. Longworth, Infections of intracardiac devices. Cardiol Clin, 2003. 21(2): p. 253–271.

[108] McGee, D.C. and M.K. Gould, Preventing complications of central venous catheterization. N Engl J Med, 2003. 348(12): p. 1123–1133.

[109] O'Donnell, A.E., et al., Pulmonary complications associated with illicit drug use: an update. CHEST J, 1995. 108(2): p. 460–463.

[110] Moreira, D., et al., Isolated pulmonary valve endocarditis in a normal heart. Rev Port Cardiol, 2012. 31(9): p. 615–617.

[111] Wong, K., et al., Clinical and radiographic spectrum of septic pulmonary embolism. Arch Dis Child, 2002. 87(4): p. 312–315.

[112] Iwasaki, Y., et al., Spiral CT findings in septic pulmonary emboli. Eur J Radiol, 2001. 37(3): p. 190–194.

[113] Sachdev, M., G.E. Peterson, and J.G. Jollis, Imaging techniques for diagnosis of infective endocarditis. Infect Dis Clin N Am, 2002. 16(2): p. 319–337.

[114] Sexton, D.J. and D. Spelman, Current best practices and guidelines: assessment and management of complications in infective endocarditis. Cardiol Clin, 2003. 21(2): p. 273–282.

[115] Bayer, A.S., et al., Diagnosis and management of infective endocarditis and its complications. Circulation, 1998. 98(25): p. 2936–2948.

[116] Moss, R. and B. Munt, Injection drug use and right sided endocarditis. Heart, 2003. 89(5): p. 577–581.

[117] Prendergast, B. and P. Tornos, Surgery for infective endocarditis: who and when? Circulation, 2010. 121(9): p. 1141.

[118] Akinosoglou, K., et al., Right-sided infective endocarditis: surgical management. Eur J Cardio-Thorac Surg, 2012. 42(3): p. 470–479.

[119] Olsson, R.A. and M.J. Romansky, Staphylococcal tricuspid endocarditis in heroin addicts. Annals Intern Med, 1962. 57(5): p. 755–762.

[120] Wang, Y.-J., et al., Liver abscess secondary to sigmoid diverticulitis: A case report. J Intern Med Taiwan, 2005. 16: p. 289–294.

[121] Rivero, A., et al., K2 serotype *Klebsiella pneumoniae* causing a liver abscess associated with infective endocarditis. J Clin Microbiol, 2010. 48(2): p. 639–641.

[122] Weng, S.-W., et al., Recurrent Klebsiella pneumoniae liver abscess in a diabetic patient followed by Streptococcus bovis endocarditis—occult colon tumor plays an important role. Jpn J Infect Dis, 2005. 58(2): p. 70–72.

[123] Katsura, M., et al., True aneurysm of the pancreaticoduodenal arteries: a single institution experience. J Gastrointest Surg, 2010. 14(9): p. 1409–1413.

[124] Brunson, J.G., Coronary embolism in bacterial endocarditis. Am J Pathol, 1953. 29(4): p. 689.

[125] Whitaker, J., et al., Successful treatment of ST elevation myocardial infarction caused by septic embolus with the use of a thrombectomy catheter in infective endocarditis. BMJ Case Rep, 2011. 2011: p. bcr0320114002.

[126] Baek, M.-J., et al., Mitral valve surgery with surgical embolectomy for mitral valve endocarditis complicated by septic coronary embolism. Eur J Cardio-Thorac Surg, 2008. 33(1): p. 116–118.

[127] Kessavane, A., et al., Septic coronary embolism in aortic valvular endocarditis. J Heart Valve Dis, 2009. 18(5): p. 572–574.

[128] Taniike, M., et al., Acute myocardial infarction caused by a septic coronary embolism diagnosed and treated with a thrombectomy catheter. Heart, 2005. 91(5): p. e34–e34.

[129] Mandell, G.L., et al., Enterococcal endocarditis: an analysis of 38 patients observed at the New York Hospital-Cornell Medical Center. Arch Intern Med, 1970. 125(2): p. 258–264.

[130] Salgado, A.V., A.J. Furlan, and T.F. Keys, Mycotic aneurysm, subarachnoid hemorrhage, and indications for cerebral angiography in infective endocarditis. Stroke, 1987. 18(6): p. 1057–1060.

[131] Guler, N., et al., Ruptured abdominal aortic aneurysm after resection of an infected cardiac myxoma. Texas Heart Inst J, 2007. 34(2): p. 233.

[132] Sandson, T.A. and J.H. Friedman, Spinal cord infarction. Report of 8 cases and review of the literature. Medicine (Baltimore), 1989. 68(5): p. 282–292.

[133] Jones, H.R., Jr. and R.G. Siekert, Neurological manifestations of infective endocarditis. Review of clinical and therapeutic challenges. Brain, 1989. 112 (Pt 5): p. 1295–1315.